A
Guide to Drugs
in Current Use

EDITED BY
PROFESSOR J. R. TROUNCE

Professor of Clinical Pharmacology
Guy's Hospital Medical School
London

MTP
MEDICAL AND TECHNICAL PUBLISHING
CO LTD · AYLESBURY
1970

Published in Great Britain by MTP
(Medical and Technical Publishing Co Ltd)
Chiltern House, Aylesbury

SBN 852 000 200

ISBN-13: 978-94-011-5898-5   e-ISBN-13: 978-94-011-5896-1
DOI: 10.1007/978-94-011-5896-1

Contents

A*

Contents

A Guide to
Drugs in Current Use

Introduction

One of the major problems which face those who are engaged in treating patients is the large number of drugs available. These drugs are often powerful agents with potential to do harm as well as good.

This book is not a treatise on therapy and the particular drug or drugs which should be used in a given clinical situation can be found elsewhere. Once however the line of treatment has been decided it is the duty of the doctor to know as much as possible about the drugs which he intends to use. It has been our aim to provide a short account of most of the drugs in current use with particular emphasis on side effects and contraindications. There is also a short review of drug interaction at the end.

In some 70,000 words it has obviously not been possible to cover every aspect of every drug and a certain amount of selection of what is considered important has had to be made. However, it is hoped that nothing of real importance has been omitted. A few references have been included where they were considered useful. These will prove useful if the reader requires a more complete knowledge of a drug. In the case of drugs not covered by a reference, one of the many large textbooks of pharmacology should be adequate. The main difficulty is with very new drugs which are not yet in standard texts and further information about them can usually only be obtained from the literature.

It will be noted that only approved names of drugs have been used. It is arguable that trade names are widely known and easier to remember. However, many drugs have more than one trade name and if these were used or even given as an alternative in the text it would lead to considerable confusion and difficulty.

Category 1

Drugs Used in Neurological Disease

THE TREATMENT OF EPILEPSY

Phenobarbitone

Pharmacological action. The drug is an effective anticonvulsant for generalised convulsive seizures and focal seizures. The neural synapse is probably its major site of action. It is thought that the drug slows or blocks cation transport of sodium and potassium across the cellular membrane and that this action damps down both excitatory and inhibitory post-synaptic potential generation. Barbiturates exert a markedly depressant effect upon repetitive activity in CNS pathways.

Therapeutic use [1]. The drug is used in the treatment of grand mal epilepsy and focal epilepsy. Temporal lobe epilepsy responds less satisfactorily. The usual starting daily intake for adults is about 100 mg per day, taken in three divided doses or in a single dose at bedtime. Daily doses are increased if seizures persist, but should rarely exceed 300 mg per day. Initial daily doses for children are smaller, usually 45 to 60 mg per day. If phenobarbitone must be discontinued after prolonged use, withdrawal should proceed slowly over a period of a week to avoid the possibility of withdrawal convulsions. However, this complication is uncommon with phenobarbitone because of its slow rate of metabolism and elimination.

Side effects and contraindications. 1. The sedative effect of the drug is a drawback. This can be circumvented by giving the total daily dose in the early evening and perhaps by medicating with central nervous system stimulants (amphetamines) during the waking hours.

2. Occasionally, for reasons as yet not clearly explained, phenobarbitone has a paradoxical exciting effect on children, the mentally retarded, and the elderly.

3. One or two per cent of patients receiving the drug develop dermatitis, which necessitates withdrawal of the drug. Rare instances of exfoliative dermatitis have been reported. The drug is contraindicated in hepatic failure, as it is normally metabolised by hepatic enzymes; in acute intermittent porphyria it may produce a precipitous and danger-

2

ous rise in the level of porphyrins which is associated with the development of symptoms of acute porphyria.

Primidone

Pharmacological action [1]. This drug is structurally closely related to phenobarbitone and its mechanism and site of action are probably the same. It is effective in the treatment of convulsive seizures refractory to other medications. However, its effectiveness against temporal lobe epilepsy and sometimes against petit mal suggests mechanisms of action additional to those of phenobarbitone.

Therapeutic use. It is used for grand mal epilepsy and temporal lobe seizures. The drug is approximately one-fifth to one-tenth as potent as phenobarbitone. The average daily dose for adults is 750 mg, and for children 150 to 250 mg.

Side effects. The effectiveness of the drug as an anticonvulsant is limited by its sedative properties. Skin rashes and leucopenia have been reported, but are rare.

Phenytoin sodium (Diphenylhydantoin, USA)

Pharmacological action. The drug suppresses local spread of epileptiform activity but it does not depress spontaneous epileptiform discharge from the epileptic focus itself. The primary action of the drug is in stabilising excitable membranes.

Therapeutic use. The drug is the most effective and widely used anticonvulsant in the treatment of generalised convulsive seizures and focal epilepsy. Therapy is usually started in the adult with 100 mg three times per day. Doses can be increased to the point of intoxication or of cessation of seizures. Lack of effect on seizures of prescribed daily doses above 500 to 600 mg suggests that the patient is not taking that amount of drug, or, in rare instances, that intestinal absorption is inadequate or that metabolism of the drug is over active. Doses above 500 mg per day are rarely necessary or tolerated.

Side effects. 1. Very few patients are hypersensitive to the drug or become intoxicated with the usual daily doses. In the few patients this may be due to a defect in the metabolism of the drug by the liver or to interference with metabolism of the drug by other drugs. In such a case reduction of dosage to 100–200 mg per day may provide adequate protection from seizures and prevent intoxication.

3

2. The features of overdosage are mainly neurological; the most striking effects are ataxia, nystagmus, dysarthria, incoordination and unsteadiness. Lethargy and drowsiness commonly occur.

3. Chronic intoxication and severe acute intoxication have resulted in Purkinje cell degeneration in the cerebellum.

4. Gum hypertrophy is common with chronic use and may be partially prevented by good dental hygiene.

5. A morbilliform rash occurs in 2–5 per cent of patients. It clears after discontinuing the drug, and does not recur when the drug is restarted.

6. Lupus erythematosus is a rare complication. When it does occur there is a positive family history of lupus erythematosus in 20 per cent of the patients.

7. Hirsutism occurs to some degree in 75 per cent of the patients who take the drug.

8. Megaloblastic anaemia occurs rarely. It is due to interference with folic acid metabolism and can be prevented by daily folic acid administration. Other blood dyscrasias are rare.

9. Hepatitis is rare. The drug should be withdrawn if it occurs.

Methoin (Mephenytoin, USA)
Pharmacological action. The drug is related chemically and pharmacologically to diphenylhydantoin. It simulates the activity of the anticonvulsant barbiturates, and it also acts as a hydantoin in preventing the tonic phase of major motor convulsions.

Therapeutic use. The drug is of value in the treatment of generalised and major motor convulsions. It is also effective to some extent in preventing temporal lobe automatisms. It has little effect on petit mal seizures, and may make them worse. The dose is 100 mg daily, increased to 600 mg in accordance with the needs of the patient.

Side effects and contraindications. The drug possesses the disagreeable characteristics of the barbiturates (sedation and lethargy) often at less than optimum therapeutic levels. As a hydantoin it is considerably more toxic than diphenylhydantoin. The most dangerous toxic effects are leukopenia, pancytopenia, agranulocytosis, and aplastic anaemia. Lymphadenopathy may occur.

Troxidone (Trimethadione, USA)
Pharmacological action. Troxidone is an anti-epileptic drug with specificity for the treatment of petit mal seizures. It is probable that troxidone

blocks the propagation of an epileptic discharge from a cortical epileptic focus to the thalamus, while the local cortical spread of the epileptiform activity is only slightly reduced, if at all.

Therapeutic use. The drug is used for the treatment of petit mal epilepsy. For an adult the dose is 900 mg daily, in divided doses, increasing to 1·8 g. daily, according to the needs of the patient. For children the dose is 300 mg. daily, in divided doses, increasing to 900 mg.

Side effects and contraindications. A frequently observed side effect is hemeralopia or night blindness. This probably represents a drug action at the ganglion layer of the retina.

Skin rashes occur with troxidone; they indicate a sensitivity reaction and their occurrence is an indication for drug withdrawal.

Bone marrow depression may occur, usually during the first year of treatment.

Nephrosis, hepatitis and lupus erythematosus have been reported.

Ethosuximide
Pharmacological action. This is the drug of choice in the treatment of petit mal and myoclonic seizures. It is extremely effective.

Therapeutic use. The adult dose is 500 mg daily, in divided doses, increasing to 2 g., according to the needs of the patient.

Side effects and contraindications. The drug is relatively non-toxic. Side effects occur infrequently, viz. gastro-intestinal upset, headache, dizziness, and skin rash. Blood changes are rare.

Sulthiame
Pharmacological action. This drug is a sulfonamide congener with weak carbonic anhydrase activity. It has reported success in the treatment of temporal lobe epilepsy, although its mode of action is not known and trials have not shown the drug to be convincingly superior to other available medications.

Therapeutic use. The drug is given for psychomotor epilepsy in doses of 200–800 mg daily.

Side effects. As the drug is a carbonic anhydrase inhibitor it may produce features of metabolic acidosis such as over-breathing. It potentiates phenobarbitone and the hydantoins, and this may account for some of its therapeutic effect. Headache, nausea, vomiting, dizziness, drowsiness, visual blurring, gastric disturbances and rarely psychoses may complicate its use.

Diazepam

Pharmacological action. This drug is thought to exert an action upon the limbic system or its connections to reduce the intensity of emotional feeling. In addition, it has an anti-epileptic effect and in particular it appears to be extremely effective in arresting status epilepticus without producing overwhelming narcosis.

Therapeutic use [2]. The chief value of the drug in epilepsy is in the control of status epilepticus. The drug is given parenterally, either in a single dose of 10 mg by slow intravenous injection, or by intravenous infusion of 100 mg over a 12-hour period.

Side effects. Weakness, drowsiness and ataxia may be produced. Long-term usage may result in habituation and very rarely in dependence. The drug may 'normalise' an abnormal E.E.G. tracing and therefore should not be given in the 10 days preceding an E.E.G. examination.

THE TREATMENT OF MIGRAINE

Ergotamine tartrate

Pharmacological action. This drug causes vasoconstriction of the cerebral vessels. It is the only drug which is sufficiently constant in effect and duration in the management of attacks of migraine.

Therapeutic use [3]. Patients vary enormously in their response to the drug; to obtain optimum results experiment is necessary in dosage and route of administration. It can be given orally, rectally, by inhalation, or by injection, and must be taken in adequate dosage as early as possible in the attack. Ideally the patient should rest in a dark room for an hour or two afterwards. The addition of caffeine is definitely advantageous; a sedative anti-emetic is added to some preparations. Taken orally ergotamine is often ineffective, and vomiting prevents its absorption. Chewing or sucking one or two tablets before the headache is well established frequently aborts the attack. The best ways of giving ergotamine are usually by suppository or inhalation, although with inhalation there is the hazard of overdosage. Some patients require injection of the drug at the very onset of an attack. Patients must be instructed not to exceed the permitted dose. Details of preparations and doses are given in the following table:

Tablets: Ergotamine   1 mg;
$\left\{\begin{array}{l}\text{Ergotamine} \ \ 1 \text{ mg} \\ \text{Caffeine} \ \ \ \ \ 100 \text{ mg}\end{array}\right.$
or
$\left\{\begin{array}{l}\text{Ergotamine} \ \ 1 \text{ mg} \\ \text{Medozine} \ \ \ 10 \text{ mg} \\ \text{Caffeine} \ \ \ \ \ 100 \text{ mg}\end{array}\right.$

1 or 2 at first sign of attack, repeated as required, $\frac{1}{2}$–1 hour later.

Solution   Dihydroergotamine 2 mg/ml
20 drops, repeated as required $\frac{1}{2}$–1 hour later.

Suppository
$\left.\begin{array}{ll}\text{Ergotamine} & 2 \text{ mg} \\ \text{Caffeine} & 100 \text{ mg} \\ \text{Belladonna} & 0\cdot25 \text{ mg} \\ \text{Isobutalyl barbituric acid} & 100 \text{ mg}\end{array}\right\}$

Medihaler   Vials: 9 mg Ergotamine/ml.
A measured dose of 0·36 mg is delivered at each operation of the aerosol.

MAXIMUM DOSES: 4 mg ERGOTAMINE DAILY; 8 mg WEEKLY

Injection: Ampoules: 0·5 mg Ergotamine/ml
0·25 mg I.M. or S.C. at onset of symptoms
Not more than 0·5 mg in the day.

Side effects and contraindications. The common side effects of ergotamine are numbness, tingling and chilling of the extremities, a rise in blood pressure, painful uterine contractions, and, particularly when it is injected, nausea and vomiting. Variability in tolerance to the drug is marked; some patients can tolerate frequent large doses, and in others extreme sensitivity may be encountered.

The contraindications to its use include peripheral vascular disease (particularly Raynaud's and Buerger's disease), hypertension, coronary, renal and hepatic insufficiency, pregnancy, and sepsis and infections which seem to sensitise to the drug. In migrainous hemiparesis the drug may prolong arterial spasm and induce a true cerebral thrombosis.

Methysergide
Pharmacological action. The exact pharmacological action of methysergide in migraine is not known. This drug is the most powerful known antagonist to serotonin; it is structurally similar to serotonin and this antagonism is possibly due to competition for similar receptors. It is therefore possible that methysergide acts by competitively inhibiting

7

the effect of serotonin on the carotid tree or by modifying its central vasomotor mechanism in the hypothalamus. However, it is quite probable that the pharmacological action of the drug may be completely independent of its ability to antagonise serotonin and bradykinin and that it is changed in the body in such a way as to acquire the long-acting, vasoconstrictor properties of ergot, or to increase the patient's sensitivity to endogenous and exogenous vasoconstrictor agents.

Therapeutic use [4]. The drug is used in the prophylaxis of migraine. 1-6 mg is used daily. A small dose of 1-2 mg is given at night for a week, during which time the patient is observed for untoward symptoms. If these do not occur the dose can be increased to a maximum of 6 mg daily. Continuous treatment for more than 6 months is undesirable without a drug-free interval for at least a month. The dosage should be decreased gradually for 2 or 3 weeks before withdrawing the drug to prevent the occurrence of a rebound phenomenon. The patient should be carefully examined at least every 3 months for the development of side effects. The prospect of serious side effects is greatly minimised when methysergide can be given intermittently for short periods only.

Side effects and contraindications. There is great individual variation in susceptibility to methysergide. Some 40 per cent of patients taking the drug experience side effects and these are so severe as to require stopping its administration in about 15 per cent.

The most common early side effects are a stimulant effect on the appetite; nausea, vomiting and diarrhoea, abdominal pain which may be due to vasoconstriction of the abdominal vasculature, peripheral oedema – probably due to constriction of veins and lymphatics; thrombophlebitis, and symptoms resulting from vasoconstriction of any artery in the body. These effects are quickly reversible when the administration of the drug is stopped.

The most important side effect of treatment with methysergide is the development of retroperitoneal fibrosis. This may develop after more than 4 months of treatment; most patients give the history of having taken the drug for many months or years. Presentation may be with low-grade fever, pain in the loins, oliguria, dysuria, and symptoms of uraemia, and confirmation is with pyelographic evidence of ureteric obstruction. About 1 per cent of patients taking the drug develop this complication; in these cases it should be withdrawn and not used again.

Methysergide is contraindicated in pregnancy, arterial and venous disease of all types, valvular heart disease, chronic pulmonary disease, impaired renal or hepatic function, peptic ulcer, and anything suggesting a diathesis of collagen disease, or a pathological tendency to fibrosis.

THE TREATMENT OF PARKINSON'S DISEASE

Artane hydrochloride (Trihexipleridyl hydrochloride, USA)
Pharmacological action. The actions of this drug on the central nervous system resemble those of the belladonna alkaloids. The evidence is that artane acts by blocking acetylcholine at certain cerebral synaptic sites.

Therapeutic use [4]. The drug is used for the symptomatic control of all forms of Parkinsonism, including the postencephalitic, arteriosclerotic, and idiopathic types. The drug favourably influences rigidity and akinesia in the majority of patients. Tremor is generally improved as well, but in some instances of severe rigidity the tremor may be accentuated when the rigidity is diminished.

The drug is virtually devoid of serious systemic toxicity.

It is the drug of choice for initial therapy of the various types of Parkinson's disease. The initial doses should be small – 1 or 2 mg twice daily, with meals. The dose is gradually increased to 2 mg three or four times daily. In some cases, the total daily dose for optimal results is 15–30 mg. The factors which determine dosage are the patient's response to therapy and his tolerance for the drug.

Side effects and contraindications. The side effects of the drug resemble those of atropine. Five to ten per cent of patients cannot tolerate fully effective doses. Side effects such as dry mouth and blurred vision are common. Overdosage produces mental confusion, delirium, agitation and hallucination. When intolerable side effects occur the dose must be reduced and if necessary another drug used along with artane, or the drug must be withdrawn in favour of another drug.

Cycrimine hydrochloride
Pharmacological action. This drug closely resembles artane hydrochloride in its action and therapeutic use.

Therapeutic use. The drug serves as a substitute for artane in the event that that agent is not well tolerated. The dose is 1·25 or 2·5 mg four times daily, initially, and it is increased according to the patient's need. The total daily dose usually does not exceed 20 mg except in post encephalitic patients, who may require as much as 45 mg daily.

Side effects. These are similar to those of artane. Large doses cause excitatory effects.

Procyclidine

Pharmacological action. This drug closely resembles artane hydrochloride in its action and therapeutic use.

Therapeutic use. The usual dose of procyclidine is 2·5 mg three times daily. This may be increased according to the tolerance of the patient to as much as 45 to 60 mg per day. The indication for the drug is as for cycrimine hydrochloride.

Side effects. These resemble those of artane.

Biperiden

Pharmacological action. The drug closely resembles artane in its pharmacological action and therapeutic use.

Therapeutic use. The drug is given as biperiden hydrochloride. The initial dose is 2 mg three or four times daily.

Side effects. Resemble those of artane.

Benztropine mesylate

Pharmacological action. This drug contains both an atropine moiety (tropine base) and an antihistaminic element (benzohydryloxy moiety). The drug possesses atropine-like as well as antihistaminic properties.

Therapeutic use. The drug may be given orally, or by intramuscular or intravenous injection. Initially, single daily doses of 0·5 to 1 mg are employed. This may be increased by daily increments of 0·5 mg until the optimum response is obtained; the maximum dose rarely exceeds 8 mg per day.

It is useful in all types of parkinsonism, and it is an effective drug to replace artane and its congeners in patients who have become tolerant to these agents. A desirable feature of the drug is its long action. The drug produces mild sedation characteristic of the antihistamines, and it is therefore an appropriate drug for patients, particularly the aged, who are adversely affected by the agents which produce excitement. Benztropine mesylate is especially effective in relieving 'frozen states'. A significant effect of the drug is the amelioration of pain secondary to muscle spasm and cramping.

Side effects. These are usually mild, and mainly associated with the anticholinergic component of the drug. Occasionally, weakness in certain muscles necessitates reduction in dosage.

Orphenadrine hydrochloride

Pharmacological action. The drug exerts a central anticholinergic action on the nervous system.

Therapeutic use. This agent reduces the rigidity of parkinsonism but it has little effect on the tremor. With favourable response there is increased muscular power and endurance. The drug produces euphoria. The initial dose is 50 mg three times daily. Total dose may be increased to 300 mg per day if necessary.

Side effects. Drowsiness is a common side effect. The peripheral anticholinergic action of the drug is relatively weak.

Chlorphenoxamine hydrochloride

The pharmacological action, therapeutic use, dosage and side effects of this drug are similar to orphenadrine. The duration of action is however slightly greater.

Ethopropazine hydrochloride

Pharmacological action. The drug is a phenothiazine derivative which possesses anticholinergic actions on the central and the peripheral nervous systems. In addition, it exerts a slight antihistaminic effect.

Therapeutic use. The initial dose is 10 mg four times daily. The dose is increased as required, and total daily doses as high as 1 g. have been employed. The drug is effective against the tremor and rigidity of parkinsonism. Sialorrhoea is well controlled.

Side effects. The side effects characteristic of anticholinergic drugs are produced by ethopropazine. Dizziness and drowsiness are common.

L-dihydroxyphenyllanine

Pharmacological action. The theoretical basis for the use of dopa in parkinsonism rests on the observation that dopamine, of which dopa is the precursor, is depleted in the corpus striatum of patients with this disease. It has been supposed that dopa administered to patients with Parkinson's disease may improve neurological function by increasing levels of dopamine in the striatum. Dopa must be used since dopamine will not pass the blood-brain barrier. It is possible that loading the central nervous system with dopa may have very much more complex and as yet obscure therapeutic effects in Parkinson's disease.

Therapeutic use [5]. Early studies indicate that most patients with idiopathic Parkinson's disease derive benefit from treatment with L-dopa. The beneficial response appears to be chiefly noticeable in the akinesia. Rigidity is improved in most patients, but there is no consistent reduction in tremor. A mild euphoriant action may occur with treatment with L-dopa but this is not thought to account for its beneficial action in more than a small minority of patients. The optimum dose lies between 3 g. and 8 g. daily.patients with post-encephalitic parkinsonism appear to respond best.

Side effects. About one-third of patients cannot tolerate a therapeutic dose of L-dopa because of nausea or vomiting. Mild nausea or vomiting is a common complication of normal therapeutic doses. This is less common or severe if the drug is taken after food. Postural hypotension and mild fall in lying systolic blood pressure have been observed. Mild intermittent abnormal movements involving the mouth, tongue, face and neck may be seen. Hypomanic and hyperactive confusional states have been described.

THE TREATMENT OF TRIGEMINAL NEURALGIA

Carbamazepine

Pharmacological action. This drug is an iminodibenzyl compound which is chemically related to imipramine. It has anticonvulsant activity.

Therapeutic use. Dose is 100 mg twice daily, gradually increasing to 200 mg three or four times daily as required. The majority of patients obtain relief within 48 hours of starting treatment.

Side effects are common. They include giddiness, nausea, anorexia, vomiting and skin rashes. Serious toxic effects have been reported; aplastic anaemia, lupus erythematosus, and the Stevens-Johnson syndrome. Adverse effects are most likely to occur when high doses of the drug are required.

References

1. Schmidt, R. P., and Wilder, B. J., *Epilepsy* (1968), Blackwell, Oxford, 141.
2. Pryse-Phillips, W., *Epilepsy* (1969), 59. John Wright, Bristol.
3. Dunlop, D., Background to migraine (1969), Report of the second migraine symposium, 72. Heinemann, London.
4. Goodman, L. S., and Gilman, A., *The Pharmacological basis of Therapeutics* (1965). Macmillan, New York, 241.
5. Godwin Austin, R. B., Tomlinson, E. B., Frears, C. C., Kok, H. W. L., *Lancet* (1969), ii, 165.'

This chapter was written by Dr P. I. Folb (Dept of Clinical Pharmacology, Guy's Hospital Medical School) and edited by Professor J. R. Trounce.

Category 2

Hypnotics

The Barbiturates

Pharmacology. The group of barbiturate hypnotics have the general formula

$$\begin{array}{ccc}
HN & \underline{\hspace{1cm}} & CO \\
| & & \diagup R_1 \\
O=C & & C \\
| & & \diagdown R_2 \\
HN & \underline{\hspace{1cm}} & CO
\end{array}$$

Substitution can occur in the R_1 and R_2 position, producing a large number of compounds. For example:

	R_1	R_2
Quinalbarbitone	$CH_2CH=CH_2$	C_5H_{11}
Amylobarbitone	C_2H_5	C_5H_{11}
Phenobarbitone	C_2H_5	Phenyl

The introduction of a phenyl group confers anticonvulsant properties and also decreases conjugation in the liver, and thus prolongs action.

This group of drugs is well absorbed from the intestinal tract and penetrates widely through the tissues. They are largely conjugated in the liver and only phenobarbitone is excreted to any degree (30 per cent) unchanged in the urine. Renal excretion is enhanced in an alkaline urine, as this increases the ionised fraction in the urine, and decreases back diffusion from the tubules to the blood [1]. With repeated dosage tolerance will develop, and it has been shown that barbiturates will induce enzymes in the liver which metabolise the drug. The enhanced production of glucuranyl transferase by barbiturates has been used in treating neonatal jaundice [2].

The effect of the very short-acting barbiturate is terminated by re-distribution of the drug – a short while after administration a major portion passes from the brain to fat and muscle.

Barbiturates produce sleep by depressing both the cortex and reticular activating system. In larger doses they produce unconsciousness and the very quick acting ones can be used as anaesthetic agents.

In hypnotic doses the barbiturates have no effect on perception of pain, and in those suffering pain they must be combined with an analgesic.

Barbiturates lower the blood pressure by reducing cardiac output [3]. This is partially due to venous pooling and perhaps also to a direct effect on the myocardium.

The respiratory centre is depressed, especially with large doses, and this is an important feature of overdosage.

Therapeutic uses. Barbiturates can be classified in terms of their duration of action.

Long Acting Group: Phenobarbitone (Phenobarbital, *USA*) is the most important. Its action is generally considered too long for a hypnotic but unlike other barbiturates it is an anticonvulsant and is used in grand mal epilepsy. The usual anticonvulsant dose is 30–60 mg two or three times daily, but the top range of dose may well produce drowsiness. The sodium salt is also available for intramuscular injection in doses of 60–200 mg in status epilepticus. It is also used as a sedative in doses of 30 mg twice daily.

Medium Acting Group: This includes the commonly used hypnotics. Various members of the group vary a little in their speed of onset and duration of action, but generally they produce sleep in about half an hour, which lasts about six hours.

Most commonly used are:

UK	USA	Dose		
Pentobarbitone	Pentobarbital	100–200 mg	very	
Quinalbarbitone	Secobarbital	50–200 mg	rapidly	
Heptobarbitone	Heptobarbital	200–400 mg	metabolised	
Amylobarbitone sodium	Amobarbital	100–200 mg	less rapidly	
Butobarbitone	Butobarbital	100–200 mg	metabolised	

The actual dose of barbiturate used will depend on the size of the patient and on any complicating factors which may modify the patient's sensitivity to the drug (see below).

Short Acting Group: This group includes thiopentone sodium (thiopental, *USA*) and hexobarbitone sodium (hexobarbital, *USA*).

They are used for short duration anaesthesia and also for induction of anaesthetics.

Contraindications and side effects. Barbiturates should not be given to those who have previously had a hypersensitivity reaction to them. Barbiturates will precipitate an acute attack of porphyria in those with this disease.

They should be used with great care if at all in those with decreased liver function or with chronic respiratory disease. In the elderly, barbiturates may produce confusion rather than sleep.

Skin rashes are the commonest side effect with barbiturates and may take a variety of forms from irritating erythemas to bullous eruptions.

The most important side effects are overdosage and dependence.

An overdose of barbiturates produces coma with respiratory depression. With very large doses there is also a falling blood pressure with circulatory, and ultimately, renal failure. The lethal dose is variable, as is the fatal blood level. In general, a blood level of more than 3·0 mg per 100 ml with a short acting barbiturate or 10 mg per 100 ml with phenobarbitone, suggests a seriously ill patient, and patients with double this level will probably require the attention of a fully equipped poisons and renal unit. It must be remembered that the effects of barbiturates will be enhanced by other CNS depressant drugs, in particular alcohol.

Dependence on barbiturates is now recognised as a serious problem [4]. Continued taking of barbiturates in doses of 600 mg daily or more causes chronic intoxication [5] with psychological dependence, weakness, dizziness, slurred speech, nystagmus and sometimes orthostatic hypotension. Withdrawal symptoms can be severe and include anxiety, weakness, and in particular, convulsions.

NON-BARBITURATE HYPNOTICS

Glutethimide

Pharmacological action. Glutethimide is related to the barbiturates but is usually called a 'non-barbiturate' hypnotic. It is fairly well absorbed from the intestinal tract and is entirely metabolised in the body. It produces sleep lasting about 6–8 hours.

Therapeutic use. Glutethimide is a useful hypnotic in doses of 250–500 mg before retiring.

Contraindications and side effects. Contraindications are similar to those for the barbiturates. Side effects are skin rashes and nausea. Rarely it may produce convulsions. Glutethimide has some cholinergic blocking effect and may interfere with bowel or bladder function. Dependence can occur.

Overdosage differs from barbiturates in that although there is some respiratory depression failing circulation with low blood pressure is a prominent feature – the pupils are also widely dilated due to the drug's anticholinergic action.

Carbromal

Pharmacological action. Carbromal is a bromine-containing derivative of urea. It is a mild, short-acting hypnotic (about four hours) and is given in doses of 300–900 mg. It can however, cause rashes which may be purpuric, and bromism can occur after prolonged use.

Chloral hydrate

Pharmacological action. Chloral hydrate is well absorbed from the intestine. In the body it is rapidly converted to trichlorethanol which is the main active substance. Trichlorethanol is inactivated by conversion to the glucuronide, and to trichloracetic acid. These products are excreted in the urine. Chloral produces sleep lasting about eight hours.

Therapeutic use. Chloral is a gastric irritant and is therefore usually given well diluted in a solution such as chloral mixture BNF (10 mls contains 1·0 g.) or as syrup of chloral hydrate U.S.P. It has an unpleasant taste. The usual adult dose is 1–2 g. but some adults may require a larger dose. It is particularly useful and safe as a hypnotic or sedative in children when the dose is 15–30 mg/kg bodyweight. It is also said to be less liable than the barbiturates to cause confusion in the elderly.

Contraindications and side effects. Chloral should not be used in patients with peptic ulcer, in those with severe liver disease or in renal failure. Chloral can occasionally cause rashes. Overdosage is rarely a serious problem.

There are a number of chloral compounds which are similar in action and uses to chloral. Unlike chloral however they are stable in tablet form and less liable to cause gastric irritation and are more palatable:

UK	USA	Dose
Dichlorphenazone		0·65–2·0 g.
Triclofos	Trichlorethylphosphate	1·0–2·0 g.
Chloral betaine		0·87–1·75 g.

The phenazone moeity of dichlorphenazone, which itself is a mild analgesic, can cause skin rashes and rarely agranulocytosis.

Ethchlorvynol
This mild hypnotic has a particularly rapid and short hypnotic effect. It has no special advantages but it is metabolised rather than excreted by the kidneys and might therefore be useful in renal failure. The dose is 250–750 mg orally.

Occasionally its use may be associated with some hang over and confusion.

Methylpentynol (Methylparafynol, USA)
This drug is a mild, short-acting hypnotic with no particular advantages. It is a liquid and is given in capsule form and may produce a rather unpleasant tasting belch. The usual dose is 250–500 mg and large doses produce a state resembling alcoholic intoxication. Rashes may occur. Methylpentynol carbamate is similar but has a more prolonged action.

Paraldehyde
Pharmacological action. Paraldehyde is a fairly powerful and rapidly acting hypnotic. It is well absorbed from the intestinal tract and from the rectum and also after intramuscular injection. It produces sleep lasting about eight hours, and is also an anticonvulsant. It is largely metabolised in the liver but about 10 per cent is excreted unchanged by the lungs.

Therapeutic use. Paraldehyde can be used as a hypnotic in doses of 3–8 ml orally, or as a 10 per cent solution in normal saline rectally. It has however largely gone out of use for it tastes unpleasant, and the patient emits a particular smell for hours after administration, from the breath, urine and sweat.

It can also be given intramuscularly in doses of 4·0 ml and repeated as required to quieten noisy patients, or in status epilepticus. By this route however it is painful, and may lead to abscess formation, so again has been largely discarded.

Contraindications and side effects. Paraldehyde is nevertheless a safe drug and side effects are rare. However, dependence can occur. Paraldehyde also changes slowly to acetic acid when stored, and bottles more than six months old should be thrown away.

Nitrazepam

Pharmacological action. Nitrazepam is a fairly quick-acting hypnotic. It is believed to depress the reticular activating system rather than the cerebral cortex. It is relatively non-toxic and considerable overdosage can occur without serious effects [6].

Therapeutic use. Nitrazepam is a useful hypnotic, as effective as the short acting barbiturates. The hypnotic action of the drug usually lasts about six hours; rarely, patients complain of some drowsiness persisting into the next day. Nitrazepam is said to be less liable to cause confusion in the elderly. The oral dose is 5–10 mg at night. In old people 2·5 mg may be sufficient.

Methaqualone

Pharmacological action. Methaqualone is a hypnotic similar in effectiveness to the barbiturates. Its action may last for 6–12 hours. The usual dose is 150–300 mg and toxic side effects are rare, but sleep may sometimes be preceded by transient paraesthesia. It is contraindicated in liver disease.

A combination of methaqualone 250 mg and diphenhydramine 25 mg per tablet is an effective hypnotic but overdosage produces drowsiness similar to that found with barbiturates. Larger doses produce a distinctive clinical picture with coma, combined with hypertonia, myoclonia and increased tendon reflexes [7].

References

1. Bunn, H. F., and Lubush, G. D., *Ann. Intern. Med.* (1965), **62**, 246.
2. Ramboer, C., Thompson, R. P. H., and Williams, R., *Lancet* (1969), **i**, 966.
3. Tuckman, J., and Shillingford, J., *Brit. J. Pharm.* (1964), **26**, 206.
4. Bewlay, I. H., *Bull Narcotics XVIII* (1966), **4**, 1.
5. Isbell, H., Altschul, S., Kornetsky, C. H., Eisenmann, A. J., Flanary, H. G., and Fraser, H. F., *Archiv. Neurol. Psychiat.* (1950), **64**, 1.
6. Matthew, H., Proudfoot, A. I., Aitkin, R. C. B., Raeburn, J. A., and Wright, N., *Brit. med. J.* (1969), **2**, 23.
7. Lawson, A. A. H., and Brown, S. S., *Scot. med. J.* (1967), **12**, 63.

This chapter was written by Professor J. R. Trounce.

The Analgesics

These can be subdivided into (i) MAJOR or narcotic analgesics and (ii) MINOR or antipyretic analgesics. For certain kinds of pain other more specific measures may be indicated, e.g. carbamazepine for trigeminal neuralgia and ergot for migraine. Details will be found in the relevant section. Certain diseases may present initially with pain as the major or only symptom, e.g. hyperparathyroidism, myxoedema and depression, and prompt diagnosis and relevant treatment may give relief. The presence and nature of a pain is frequently of diagnostic help, and the administration of an analgesic should not, wherever possible, precede or overshadow history-taking, examination and diagnosis.

THE MAJOR OR NARCOTIC ANALGESICS

Opium was the earliest source of all narcotic analgesics. All the analgesic alkaloids (e.g. morphine, codeine and thebaine) were found to be phenanthrene derivatives, whereas other alkaloids (e.g. papaverine and narcotine) were inactive as analgesics (see table 1). Other semi-synthetic and synthetic substances have since been developed and used as analgesics, yet despite wide chemical differences the pharmacological actions of all the major analgesics are very similar. For this reason morphine will be taken as the central drug of this group and discussed in some detail; the actions of the other drugs being described in relation to it.

The narcotic antagonists will also be included in this section as they are closely related to the narcotic analgesics.

Morphine
Pharmacological action. A powerful analgesic and narcotic having various stimulating and depressant actions on the nervous system. Centrally it produces euphoria and depresses the cortex, thalamus, cerebellum, respiratory and cough centres. It stimulates the vagus, vomiting centre and spinal cord and also causes constriction of the pupil. Increased ADH secretion reduces the urine output and if hypercapnia develops intra-

Table 1	The opiates	
Useful analgesics	Related drugs with other uses	

Phenanthrene Derivatives	
Morphine	Apomorphine (emetic)
Diamorphine	Ethyl morphine (eye-drops)
Papaveretum	Nalorphine*
Hydromorphone	Thebaine (not used)
Oxymorphone	
Metopon	
Codeine	
Pholcodine	
Dihydrocodeine	
Hydrocodone	
Oxycodone	
Benzylisoquinoline Alkaloids	
	Papaverine (vasodilator)

* Narcotic Antagonist.

cranial pressure may be increased. Peripherally, morphine reduces secretions and increases tone in involuntary muscle. The latter effect is most marked in the muscle and sphincters of the gastro-intestinal and biliary tracts and similar effects have been described in the urinary tract. Skin vessels are dilated and there is increased sweating.

Tolerance develops within 2-3 weeks of continuous use, chiefly in relation to its depressant actions. Physical dependence may begin even earlier leading to a withdrawal syndrome on stopping the drug. If use of the drug is prolonged overt addiction may develop.

Morphine is metabolised in the liver and excreted chiefly into the urine but also into the gut via the bile. Its analgesic effect is maximal at about 1 hour and lasts for 3-4 hours.

Therapeutic uses. Morphine sulphate is the most frequently used preparation for oral or parenteral use but other salts are available:

Oral preparations:	Morphine sulphate
	Morphine hydrochloride
Parenteral preparations:	Morphine sulphate
	Morphine tartrate
	Morphine acetate

The dose for all these preparations is roughly the same and is usually 10–15 mg. Absorption from the gastrointestinal tract is often unreliable and subcutaneous or intramuscular injection is more effective. Morphine can also be given as a slow intravenous injection.

It is used to relieve pain which is not amenable to the milder analgesics and is of particular value when this is associated with anxiety and restlessness. Its use in patients suffering from haemorrhage, trauma or shock, who are not troubled by pain, is of doubtful merit in view of the well-documented tendency for morphine to lower the blood pressure. However, it is difficult to deny its good effect when given to patients with gastro-intestinal haemorrhage and other factors may play a part here. It relieves the dyspnoea of cardiac asthma and is also used to suppress unwanted coughing, to control diarrhoea and as a premedication (with hyoscine or atropine) before surgery.

The euphoriant effect is used in the management of terminal disease and where this is associated with severe pain chlorpromazine produces a useful synergistic effect as well as having a mild anti-emetic action. In cases where respiratory depression or undue somnolence becomes a problem an analeptic such as amiphenazole (q.v.) may be used with morphine to good effect.

Contraindications and side effects. Morphine should not be used in the presence of respiratory depression, cyanosis, obstructive airways disease, hepatic insufficiency, acute alcoholism, toxic confusional states, convulsive disorders or raised intracranial pressure. It is unwise to give it alone for cholecystitis, biliary disorders, pancreatitis or diverticulitis, but increased smooth muscle activity can be offset by combination with propantheline [1]. It is badly tolerated by patients with myxoedema and the elderly and debilitated. Its action is enhanced by mono-amine oxidase inhibitors, neostigmine, chlorpromazine, barbiturates and alcohol. Potentiation occurs with hypotensive agents.

Side effects include: nausea and vomiting (especially if not resting in bed), constipation, tremors, restlessness, insomnia and rarely convulsions. Itching and urticaria occur as well as other rashes. Hypotension which may be postural is usually mild but is often pronounced when the drug is given to patients following myocardial infarction. Toxic doses produce respiratory depression, cyanosis, hypotension, pinpoint pupils and coma. These effects are best treated by an injection of one of the specific antagonists nalorphine or levallorphan (see below).

Diamorphine (Heroin, USA)

Pharmacological action. Slightly more potent than morphine. It has an earlier onset and shorter duration of action (about two hours). It more readily produces euphoria, is a powerful anti-tussive and respiratory depressant but is probably less likely to cause vomiting or constipation.

Therapeutic uses. It may be given as an elixir or linctus in a dose of 5–10 mg or by injection in a dose of 3–6 mg initially. It is not available in some countries because of the problem of addiction. It is favoured by some for the pain of acute myocardial infarction, but it has a similar effect on the blood pressure as morphine, and a recent study [2] suggests that pentazocine (see below) may be a better choice. It is most often used for terminal disease and occasionally for post-operative analgesia and sedation.

Contraindications and side effects. As morphine; it has often been thought to be more addictive but this point is still debated.

Papaveretum (total extract of opium)

Pharmacological action. Very similar to morphine which forms most of the active part of this preparation. However it is better tolerated and is said to cause less respiratory depression and vomiting.

Therapeutic use. As morphia. Dose: 10–20 mg orally or I.M.

Contraindications and side effects. As morphine.

Hydromorphone

Pharmacological action. Very similar to morphine, being slightly more potent and having a shorter duration of action.

Therapeutic use. As morphine. Dose: 2–5 mg orally; 2 mg by injection.

Contraindications and side effects. As morphine.

Oxymorphone

Pharmacological action. Slightly more potent than morphia and producing more euphoria, respiratory depression, nausea and vomiting.

Therapeutic use. Dose: 5–10 mg orally; 1·5–5 mg I.M. or S.C.

Metopon

Pharmacological action. A narcotic analgesic about twice as potent as morphine but in all other respects the same. Dose: 3–6 mg.

Codeine

Pharmacological action. Analgesic but much less potent than morphine. It is a mild hypnotic but does not depress the respiratory centre or constipate as much as morphine. It is an effective cough suppressant. Little of it is metabolised in the body, most appearing in the urine.

Therapeutic uses. It is used as the hydrochloride, phosphate or sulphate and the dose for all three salts is 10–60 mg. It is taken as a tablet, linctus or I.M. injection. It is most useful for the control of less severe pain, unwanted cough and diarrhoea. It does show a synergistic action with aspirin and is often prepared in combination with the antipyretic analgesics.

Contraindications and side effects. Less than morphine. Overdosage gives a different picture consisting of narcosis often preceded by exhilaration and excitement and followed by convulsions. Nausea and vomiting are prominent, the pupils constrict and there is a tachycardia.

Pholcodine

Pharmacological action. A derivative of morphine with almost no analgesic action. It does not suppress respiration but is an effective cough suppressant.

Dihydrocodeine

Pharmacological action. It has a shorter duration of action and is less potent than morphine. Is as good a cough suppressant as codeine.

Therapeutic use. Preparations:

Dihydrocodeine phosphate – dose 10–30 mg
Dihydrocodeine bitartrate – dose 10–60 mg

It can be given as a linctus, tablet, I.M. or S.C. injection. It has few side effects; contraindications as morphine.

Hydrocodone

Pharmacological action. Intermediate in action between morphine and codeine. It is chiefly used as a cough suppressant.

Therapeutic use. It is used as the phosphate, hydrochloride or acid tartrate. The dose for each is 5–15 mg orally but it can also be given as a S.C. injection.

Oxycodone

Pharmacological action. A moderately strong analgesic, slightly more potent and possibly more addicting than codeine.

Therapeutic use. Preparations:

Oxycodone Hydrochloride – dose 5–30 mg orally; 5 mg by injection

Oxycodone Pectinate – dose I.M. 10–20 mg

The latter acts for much longer (up to 10 hours).

Contraindications and side effects. As morphine.

Nalorphine

Pharmacological action. It is a specific narcotic analgesic antagonist reducing or abolishing most of the actions of morphine and all the major analgesics. It does not antagonise the depressant effect on the cough centre and hence there is little evidence of antagonism with pholcodine and other anti-tussives which have little analgesic effect. It acts within a few seconds of intravenous injection, increasing the rate and volume of respiration and can awaken a patient from a narcotic state. It reverses the rise in biliary pressure and miosis but has similar analgesic properties to morphine. It is not effective in reversing depression produced by barbiturates, cyclopropane or ether.

Therapeutic uses. Dose: 5–10 mg I.V. as either the hydrochloride or hydrobromide. It is used particularly to treat overdosage with narcotic analgesics and in severe cases much larger doses may be required [3]. It has also been used in a test for narcotic analgesic addiction in which the reversing effect on pupil size is noted. If given to an addict it will precipitate withdrawal symptoms.

It is also used to prevent respiratory depression in the newborn. It can be given I.V. 10 mg to the mother 10 minutes before delivery or injected directly into the umbilical vein immediately after birth (0·25–1 mg).

Table 2	Phenylheptylamine derivatives	
Useful analgesics	Related drugs with other uses
Methadone	
Phenadoxone	
Propoxyphene (d-propoxyphene)	l-Propoxyphene (anti-tussive)
Dextromoramide	
Dipipanone	

Contraindications and side effects. If given on its own it may cause respiratory depression and disturbing psychotic effects. In addicts to morphine and its derivatives it will produce withdrawal symptoms. Side effects include drowsiness, irritability, miosis, nausea, pallor, sweating and hypotension.

Methadone

Pharmacological action. A potent analgesic similar to morphine but with less sedative effect and a longer duration of action. It is more reliably absorbed from the gastro-intestinal tract.

Therapeutic use. Dose: orally 5–10 mg; I.M. 5–10 mg; linctus 1–2 mg doses. It is not used intravenously. It is useful for severe pain and unproductive cough. It is not suitable as a premedication unless combined with a short-acting barbiturate or hyoscine. It has been used in the rehabilitation of morphine and heroin addicts as withdrawal from it is less unpleasant, probably because of its longer duration of action.

Contraindications and side effects. As with morphine nausea, vomiting, dizziness, respiratory depression and constriction of the pupils occur, although it less readily produces constipation. It may lower the blood pressure and children tolerate it poorly. It is not recommended for use in obstetrics as it significantly depresses foetal respiration.

Phenadoxone

Pharmacological action. An effective analgesic with a mild hypnotic effect. It reduces smooth muscle activity and does not cause constipation in normal doses. Orally it acts within 15–30 minutes and lasts for 1–3 hours. When used parenterally there may be considerable irritation at injection sites. It is not used intravenously.

Therapeutic use. Dose: orally 10–30 mg; I.M. or S.C. 5–15 mg.

Contraindications and side effects. As for methadone.

Propoxyphene

Pharmacological action. It is chemically similar to methadone but is only a mild analgesic having a similar onset, duration of action and potency to codeine. It is not anti-tussive.

Therapeutic use. Dose: 30–60 mg orally. It is used for mild to moderate pain associated with chronic and recurrent disease. It is often combined with aspirin or paracetamol for this purpose.

Contraindications and side effects. Nausea and vomiting occur less than with codeine although it does constipate as much. In large doses it causes drowsiness, dizziness, general excitement, mental confusion, twitching, respiratory depression, convulsions and coma. Local irritation occurs if given subcutaneously. It is only mildly addictive but can block the withdrawal effects of morphine and is antagonised by nalorphine.

Dextromoramide

Pharmacological action. A strong analgesic, slightly more powerful than morphine and with a similar duration of action. It is well absorbed by mouth.

Therapeutic use. Preparations: alone or as the acid tartrate (5 mg dextromoramide ≡ 6·9 mg D. acid tartrate). Dose: 5–20 mg orally or I.M. It may also be given by S.C. or I.V. injection or administered rectally.

Contraindications and side effects. As for morphine but respiratory depression is not evident with oral therapeutic doses.

Dipipanone

Pharmacological action. A potent analgesic of similar strength to morphine with a more rapid onset but a similar duration of action. There is less respiratory depression and it is effective orally.

Therapeutic use. Dose: 25–50 mg S.C. or I.M. Oral tablets of 10 mg are usually combined with cyclizine 30 mg.

Table 3	Phenylpiperidine derivatives
Useful analgesics	Related drugs with other uses
Pethidine or Meperidine	Diphenoxylate (costive)
Alphaprodine	
Anileridine	
Piminidone	
Fentanyl	
Phenoperidine	
Ethoheptazine	

Pethidine (Meperidine, *USA*)
Pharmacological action. An effective analgesic but less potent and with about half the duration of action of morphine. It is only a mild sedative, euphoria is less marked and dysphoric sensations are more likely to occur. It does not affect the size of the pupil in therapeutic doses and is a poor cough suppressant. It does not cause constipation but its effect on smooth muscle is similar to morphine. It reduces the severity of labour pains without diminishing the force of uterine contraction but like most other major analgesics it prolongs labour.

Therapeutic uses. Dose: orally 50–100 mg; S.C. or I.M. 25–100 mg and I.V. 25–50 mg. It is used as an alternative to morphine to relieve pain; for obstetric analgesia and in conjunction with barbiturates or hyoscine to produce obstetric amnesia. It is also used commonly for pre- and post-operative medication. Pethidine (50 mg) has been combined with levallorphan tartrate (0·625 mg) as an injection. This was primarily designed for use in obstetrics but is only of marginal benefit. In view of its effect on smooth muscle it should be given with propantheline for the treatment of visceral colic [1].

Contraindications and side effects. Nausea and vomiting are as frequent as with comparable doses of morphine but constipation is less. The blood pressure may fall after I.V. administration and this is especially noticeable in patients with acute myocardial infarction [4]. Pethidine can cause excitement and dysphoria especially with overdosage when in-co-ordination, tremor, convulsions, respiratory depression and coma may supervene. Its action is potentiated by mono-amine oxidase inhibitors and phenothiazines. There is a danger of addiction.

Alphaprodine
Pharmacological action. It has a similar potency and action to pethidine but is more rapid in onset and of shorter duration. Given subcutaneously and with an adequate peripheral circulation it will have an analgesic effect within 5 minutes lasting for about 2 hours.

Therapeutic uses. Dose: S.C. 20–60 mg and I.V. 20–30 mg. It is used chiefly in obstetrics and for premedication and minor surgical procedures.

Contraindications and side effects. Dizziness, itching and sweating occur but nausea, vomiting and respiratory depression are less likely than with morphine. However, it will cause depression of foetal respiration if given within 2 hours of delivery.

Anileridine

Pharmacological action. Similar but less potent than morphine. It is rapidly absorbed by mouth and acts more quickly and for a shorter time than morphine.

Therapeutic uses. Preparations: orally anileridine hydrochloride dose 25 mg; S.C. or I.V. anileridine phosphate dose 25–50 mg. It is used as a shorter acting analgesic especially as a premedication and in obstetrics.

Contraindications and side effects. Similar to morphine but it tends to cause more restlessness and less nausea, vomiting and constipation.

Fentanyl

Pharmacological action. A very potent analgesic with a rapid onset and brief duration of action. It causes respiratory depression and has an emetic effect.

Therapeutic uses. Dose: 0·1–0·6 mg I.V. It has been primarily used in association with tranquillizers such as triperidol and droperidol to produce brief surgical anaesthesia especially in young, old and debilitated patients. They block the emetic effect and the general effects are antagonised by nalorphine.

Contraindications and side effects. As morphine.

Phenoperidine

Pharmacological action. A potent analgesic which in large doses produces sedation and respiratory suppression.

Therapeutic uses. I.M. or I.V. 0·5–1 mg for analgesia; 2–5 mg where respiratory depression is desired. It is used in similar situations to fentanyl in combination with a 'neuroleptic' agent, e.g. droperidol (q.v.) to produce surgical anaesthesia. It is of particular value for sedation during artificial ventilation.

Contraindications and side effects. As morphine.

Ethoheptazine

Pharmacological action. An analgesic of equivalent strength to codeine. It is not anti-tussive or a respiratory suppressant and does not sedate. It acts within 30 minutes and lasts for 4–5 hours.

Therapeutic uses. Dose: 75–150 mg orally. It is used chiefly in conjunction with aspirin or paracetamol.

Contraindications and side effects. Similar to morphine but appears not to be addictive.

Table 4	Morphinans and Benzmorphans	
	Useful analgesics	Related drugs with other uses
Morphinans	Levorphanol (l-methorphan)	d-Methorphan (anti-tussive) Levallorphan*
Benzmorphans	Phenazocine Pentazocine	

* Narcotic antagonist.

Levorphanol

Pharmacological action. A potent analgesic similar to morphine but causing less drowsiness. It is as effective by mouth as it is by injection.

Therapeutic uses. Dose: orally 1·5–4·5 mg; I.M. or S.C. 2–4 mg and I.V. 1–1·5 mg. It is used as an alternative to morphine and can be used for premedication (2 mg S.C.) with atropine or hyoscine.

Contraindications and side effects. As morphine.

Levallorphan

Pharmacological action. A narcotic antagonist having similar effects to nalorphine but with a greater potency and longer duration of action. Small doses antagonise the respiratory depression of narcotic drugs – larger doses also antagonising the analgesic effect.

Therapeutic uses. Dose: 1–2 mg I.V. with further doses as necessary. It is often used to reverse respiratory depression in the newborn when it is given to the mother (1–2 mg) 10 minutes before delivery or directly into the umbilical vein (0·05–0·25 mg) of the infant.

Contraindications and side effects. As for nalorphine.

Phenazocine

Pharmacological action. An analgesic of similar potency and actions to morphine. It is less sedative and may cause less respiratory depression.

Therapeutic uses. Dose: orally 5 mg; I.M. or I.V. 1–4 mg. It may be superior for obstetric use but otherwise has been used as an alternative to morphine.

Contraindications and side effects. Similar to morphine but usually less marked. Facial pruritus may follow I.V. injection.

Pentazocine

Pharmacological action. This drug was developed as an antagonist to phenazocine and was found to be a powerful analgesic itself of a similar potency to morphine. It is also sedative and does depress respiration when given parenterally. However it appears to be much less addictive and does not lower the blood pressure unlike most of the other strong analgesics.

Therapeutic use. Dose: orally 25–100 mg; S.C. or I.M. 30–60 mg and I.V. 20–30 mg. It can be used as an alternative to morphine and is probably the drug of choice for acute myocardial infarction. A recent study [2] showed that in a comparison with morphine, diamorphine methadone and pethidine it was the only drug which did not tend to lower the blood pressure. Other side effects were much the same for all these drugs.

Contraindications and side effects. Similar to morphine apart from its low addiction potential. There have been several reports of transient but disturbing hallucinations. It is not antagonised by nalorphine and it is recommended that methyl phenidate (see below) be given as an antidote instead.

Table 5 Equivalent doses of the major analgesics* (in mg)

Morphine	10	Dextromoramide	5–7·5
Diamorphine	5	Dipipanone	20–25
Hydromorphone	2	Pethidine/Meperidine	75
Oxymorphone	1	Alphaprodine	40–60
Metopon	3·5	Anileridine	30–40
Codeine	120	Piminidone	7·5–10
Dihydrocodeine	60	Phenoperidine	1·5
Oxycodone	10–15	Levorphanol	3
Methadone	10	Phenazocine	2–3
Phenadoxone	10–20	Pentazocine	30

*These doses represent that dose which when given subcutaneously produces an analgesic effect approximately equivalent to 10 mg. subcutaneous morphine.

THE MINOR ANALGESICS AND
ANTI-INFLAMMATORY AGENTS

Nearly all share analgesic, anti-pyretic and anti-rheumatic (anti-inflammatory) properties. These drugs are free of addiction potential, although patients can become habituated to their use. Their exact site of action is still not entirely clear. Vasodilation, whether produced centrally or peripherally, causes much of the antipyretic activity. The analgesia may originate centrally or may be due to a direct effect on pain receptors. A direct antagonism of various chemical mediators of inflammation may explain most of the anti-inflammatory effect.

THE SALICYLATES

Acetylsalicylic acid (aspirin)

Pharmacological action. An effective minor analgesic with considerable antipyretic and anti-inflammatory properties. In large doses it is urico-suric. In smaller doses it causes uric acid retention. It also has a mild hypoglycaemic and hypoprothrombinaemic action. It is rapidly meta-bolised to salicyclic acid which is probably responsible for most of its effects. Both acids are excreted rapidly in the urine and the more so if this is kept alkaline. Its effect lasts for about 4 hours.

Therapeutic uses. Dose: 300–1,200 mg orally. It is the most effective and useful of the minor analgesics and is used for all kinds of less severe pain, e.g. headache, neuralgia, rheumatic and muscle pains. It is of particular use for acute and chronic rheumatism. In these conditions doses of up to 4–8 g. a day are used, although in the chronic situation much less will often suffice. It has been used for gout but is inferior to the other uricosuric agents.

Contraindications and side effects. Gastric irritation is the commonest problem and may be accompanied by occult blood loss. Occasionally frank haematemesis and melaena occur. With larger doses, dizziness, tinnitus, deafness, sweating, nausea and vomiting may develop. In sensitive patients salicylates may precipitate attacks of asthma, angio-neurotic oedema and other allergy. Therapeutic doses produce minor platelet abnormalities and long-term use has caused pancytopenia [5]. Toxic doses cause hyperthermia, hyperventilation, excitement, coma and convulsions. Complex and changing acid-base disturbances also accompany overdosage. Salicylates should not be given to patients

31

having a history of dyspepsia or peptic ulceration, known sensitivity, asthma or severe renal disease.

Other preparations have been made to try and overcome the irritant effect on the stomach, e.g. aluminium acetylsalicylate and calcium acetylsalicylate. The latter is more soluble, better absorbed and less irritant than acetylsalicylic acid. It is the usual form of 'Soluble Aspirin', containing acetylsalicylic acid, calcium carbonate and citric acid, which on dissolving gives a solution of calcium acetylsalicylate. Aloxiprin is a polymeric condensation product of aluminium hydroxide and acetylsalicylic acid and is also better tolerated.

Various forms of buffered aspirin have been developed but they have little advantage over calcium aspirin. Enteric-coated preparations also cause less gastric irritation but absorption takes much longer and they are more suited to long term regular use.

Aspirin is often combined with other minor analgesics and Aspirin Compound or A.P.C. is one of the most used preparations. It contains approximately 230 mg aspirin with 150 mg phenacetin and 30 mg caffeine. Sometimes codeine is added or used as an alternative.

Sodium salicylate
Pharmacological action. Similar to aspirin but less analgesic and a more effective antipyretic. It is more irritant to the stomach.

Therapeutic uses. Dose: 600–2000 mg. It has been used for acute rheumatic fever in doses of 5–10 g. daily, but aspirin is more suitable for rheumatoid arthritis in view of its greater analgesic activity.

Contraindications and side effects. As aspirin.

PARA-AMINOPHENOL DERIVATIVES

Paracetamol (Acetaminophen, *USA*)
Pharmacological action. An effective analgesic and antipyretic of similar potency to aspirin. It has less anti-inflammatory activity, less side effects and does not cause gastric irritation. It is not uricosuric.

Therapeutic uses. Dose: 500–1000 mg as tablets or elixir. It is used widely for all kinds of mild pain and is the drug of choice when aspirin is contraindicated. It is contained in many combined analgesic preparations.

Contraindications and side effects. These are few and rarely troublesome. It is still not certain whether paracetamol can cause the same kind of renal damage as phenacetin when taken in high dosage over long periods. Liver damage may occur with over-dosage.

Phenacetin (acetophenetidin)

Pharmacological action. Similar to paracetamol. Most of its action is due to the formation of paracetamol in vivo.

Therapeutic use. Dose: 300–600 mg. It is a common constituent of analgesic combinations.

Contraindications and side effects. Its toxic effects are similar to acetanilide (see below) and are due to small amounts of aniline being formed. This may cause methaemoglobinaemia and a haemolytic anaemia. If large amounts of phenacetin are taken over a long period serious renal damage in the form of papillary necrosis and chronic interstitial nephritis may ensue. It seems that upwards of a kilogramme of phenacetin has to be ingested before this occurs but the changes may be reversible [6]. More recently the development of transitional-cell tumours of the renal pelvis has been implicated [7].

Acetanilide

Pharmacological action. As with the case of phenacetin its action is very largely due to the formation of paracetamol by the liver.

Therapeutic uses. Dose: 120–300 mg. It used to be included in most headache powders but has latterly been replaced because of its toxicity.

Contraindications and side effects. Toxicity is chiefly due to the liberation of aniline which causes methaemoglobinaemia. Large doses produce cyanosis, cardiovascular depression and collapse.

PYRAZOLONE DERIVATIVES

Phenazone (Antipyrine, USA)

Pharmacological action. An effective minor analgesic having a more, rapid and transient action than phenacetin, although like the other drugs in this group it is more potent than the salicylates. It is anti-pyretic and anti-inflammatory and in large doses uricosuric. Like the other uricosuric agents it may cause uric acid retention in low dosage.

Therapeutic uses. Dose: 300–600 mg. It is used as an alternative to aspirin and forms part of many combined remedies.

Contraindications and side effects. Rashes are common and some types of erythematous eruption leave residual pigmentation. Methaemoglobinaemia and cyanosis is a rare complication. Toxic doses produce nausea, fainting and collapse. Prolonged administration has led to agranulo-cytosis. It is nevertheless one of the least toxic drugs of this group.

Aminopyrine (Amidopyrine, USA)
Pharmacological action and side effects. In action it resembles phenazone but this drug has been withdrawn from general use because of the high incidence of agranulocytosis.

Phenylbutazone
Pharmacological action. It is analgesic, antipyretic, anti-inflammatory and uricosuric. It is hydroxylated in vivo to form oxyphenbutazone.

Therapeutic uses. Dose: orally 200–400 mg daily in divided doses, taken with food or milk. It can also be given I.M. in a dose of 600 mg (prepared with xylocaine) and rectally as 250 mg suppositories. It is used particularly for arthritic pain in association with rheumatoid arthritis, osteo-arthritis, ankylosing spondylitis, psoriasis and gout.

Contraindications and side effects. Untoward reactions are common. They include nausea, stomatitis, epigastric pain, diarrhoea, vertigo and oedema. The latter is due to sodium retention and may be offset by a low salt diet or a diuretic. Reactivation of peptic ulcers with perfora-tion, haematemesis and melaena may occur. Less often agranulocytosis, thrombocytopenia, aplastic anaemia and a macrocytic anaemia res-ponding to folic acid have occurred and a possible link with leukaemia is still uncertain. Hepatitis and acute renal failure have also been described.

Severe hypoprothrombinaemia occurs in people who are also being treated with coumarin anticoagulants and this may give rise to serious complications [8]. This effect is due to competitive binding of these drugs to plasma albumin.

Phenylbutazone should not be given to patients with known cardiac, liver or renal disease, or to those with a history of peptic ulceration, blood dyscrasia or allergy. It should not be used with gold salts.

Oxyphenbutazone
Pharmacological action and uses. A derivative of phenylbutazone with similar effects and uses. It is less effective in relieving stiffness or pain in rheumatoid arthritis or ankylosing spondylitis, but it is better tolerated. Dose: 300–600 mg daily in divided doses, taken with meals.

Contraindications and side effects. Similar to phenylbutazone but less severe.

Sulphinpyrazone

Pharmacological action and uses. A marked uricosuric agent with little direct analgesic or anti-inflammatory effect. It has been used for chronic gout in an initial dose of 50 mg q.d.s. with meals. This is increased to 500 mg daily over a period of a week and reduced to about 200 mg daily when controlled.

Contraindications and side effects. Gastro-intestinal symptoms occur but are less severe than with phenylbutazone and blood dyscrasias are rare. It should not be used in the presence of impaired renal function or peptic ulceration. Salicylates reduce its effect.

Nifenazone

Pharmacological action and uses. A pyrazolone chemically resembling amidopyrine, having analgesic, antipyretic and anti-inflammatory effects. It is inferior to phenylbutazone or oxyphenbutazone. Dose: orally 250–500 mg 1, 2 or 3 times daily. 400 mg suppositories are available for rectal use.

Contraindications and side effects. Gastro-intestinal symptoms may occur and in view of its chemical relationships blood dyscrasias are a possibility.

Phenyramidol

Pharmacological action, uses and side effects. A moderate analgesic which like phenylbutazone can cause serious hypoprothrombinaemia in patients on anticoagulant therapy. Dose: 200–400 mg. It may also cause nausea, dyspepsia, drowsiness, pruritis and skin rashes. It is contraindicated in patients having salicylate sensitivity.

QUINOLINE DERIVATIVES

Cinchophen and Neocinchophen

Pharmacological action and uses. Both these extracts from quinine or cinchona bark are analgesic and antipyretic and of similar potency to the salicylates. Neocincophen is more uricosuric and they were both used for chronic gout although more effective agents are now available. Dose: 200–500 mg.

Contraindications and side effects. Similar to the salicylates. In addition even therapeutic doses can cause hepatitis.

COLCHICINE DERIVATIVES

Colchicine

Pharmacological action. An alkaloid from meadow saffron which is analgesic for acute gout. It is also anti-mitotic but has little effect in leukaemia, although demecolcine (see below) has been used for leukaemia.

Therapeutic uses. Doses for acute gout: 1 mg stat. followed by 0·5 mg 2-hourly until pain ceases or vomiting or diarrhoea develops.

Contraindications and side effects. Stomatitis, nausea, vomiting, abdominal pain, and diarrhoea. It should be avoided in the old and feeble and in those with gastrointestinal disorders.

AN INDOLE DERIVATIVE

Indomethacin

Pharmacological action. This indole derivative is an effective analgesic, antipyretic and anti-inflammatory agent of value in acute gout and various forms of arthritis [9]. It is not recommended as a general analgesic.

Therapeutic uses. Dose: orally 25–50 mg two or three times daily. It can also be used as 100 mg suppositories. For acute gout 50 mg is recommended orally followed by 25 mg 6-hourly.

Side effects. These are frequent but usually less serious than those found with phenylbutazone. They include dizziness, headache, vertigo, drowsiness, confusion, psychiatric disturbances, anorexia, nausea, vomiting, dyspepsia, diarrhoea, gastro-intestinal bleeding and corneal and retinal changes which are usually reversible. Pruritus, rashes and oedema also occur and a reversible leucopenia has been described in patients with rheumatoid arthritis. Deaths have occurred in children treated with indomethacin and it is now only recommended for adult use.

THE FENAMATES

Mefenamic acid

Pharmacological action. A derivative of anthranilic acid which is analgesic, antipyretic and anti-inflammatory. Its analgesic effect is greater than aspirin or paracetamol and roughly equivalent to codeine. Its anti-inflammatory activity is less powerful than phenylbutazone. Its effect comes on 1 hour after an oral dose and lasts for up to 6 hours.

Therapeutic uses. Dose: 250–500 mg orally. It is used as a general analgesic as well as supplementing other measures used for arthritic pain.

Contraindications and side effects. Diarrhoea is the most common side effect but is usually reversible. Reversible leucopenia, haemolytic anaemia and maculopapular rashes have been described. Gastric irritation occurs but is much less frequent or troublesome than with aspirin. Elevation of the blood urea may occur and renal papillary necrosis has been described in animal studies.

Flufenamic acid

Pharmacological action. Similar to mefenamic acid but less analgesic and antipyretic and more anti-inflammatory. For further information see [10].

Therapeutic use. Dose: 100–200 mg t.d.s. It is most useful for arthritic pain.

Contraindications and side effects. Also tends to cause diarrhoea in some patients but so far few other side effects have been described.

PHENYLALKANOIC ACID DERIVATIVES

Ibuprofen

Pharmacological action. This is the propionic acid derivative of an earlier substance, Ibufenac (p-isobutylphenylacetic acid) which was withdrawn because of the development of jaundice as a side effect. These substances have analgesic, antipyretic and anti-inflammatory activity. Its potency is comparable to aspirin. Ibuprofen unlike ibufenac is not concentrated in the liver and does not cause jaundice.

Therapeutic uses. Dose: 200 mg t.d.s. It is recommended for arthritic pain and particularly for those intolerant to salicylates.

Contraindications and side effects. These seem to be few and although it may occasionally cause dyspepsia it so far does not seem to aggravate peptic ulcers. Pending full assessment it is best avoided in patients with any abnormality of liver function.

GOLD

Sodium aurothiomalate, aurothioglucose and aurothioglycanide.

Pharmacological action and uses. These three preparations will be considered collectively. Their action is uncertain but they have a long-lasting effect on rheumatoid arthritis, especially in the early stages. Gold is ineffective in other kinds of arthritis.

Dose: after a test dose of 10 mg I.M., weekly injections increasing by an increment of 10 mg up to 50 mg are given, usually up to a total dose of 1 g. although injections may be continued indefinitely, preferably at a reduced dose. The dosage required with aurothioglycanide may be a little higher.

Contraindications and side effects. Toxic effects occur in at least 30 per cent of cases and include pruritus, urticaria, purpura, dermatitis which may exfoliate, stomatitis which may ulcerate and less commonly thrombocytopenia, aplastic anaemia, hepatic and renal damage, peripheral neuropathy and an encephalopathy may develop. The urine should be examined for protein before each injection and blood counts made every 2–3 weeks. Gold therapy should be stopped as soon as any toxic effect appears. Serious toxic effects should be treated with dimercaprol (q.v.). Corticosteroids may be useful, especially for a severe dermatitis.

Gold should not be used in the presence of known renal or hepatic damage, anaemia, blood dyscrasias, skin diseases or any serious illness.

ANTIMALARIALS

Chloroquine phosphate and Hydroxychloroquine sulphate
Pharmacological action. Their mode of action is unknown. They have a beneficial effect in up to 50 per cent of cases of rheumatoid arthritis.

Therapeutic use. Doses: chloroquine phosphate – orally 250–750 mg daily initially, and 150 mg daily for maintenance.

Hydroxychloroquine sulphate – orally 800–1,200 mg daily initially and 200 mg daily for maintenance.

Contraindications and side effects. Toxic effects include nausea, vomiting, dizziness, diarrhoea and blurring of vision. After continued use bleached hair, rashes, corneal opacities and retinal degeneration may develop. The latter may be irreversible.

During treatment a six-monthly ophthalmic examination is mandatory in order to detect presymptomatic corneal or retinal damage. Eighth nerve damage also occurs. These drugs should not be given during pregnancy.

CORTICOSTEROIDS

Some of these agents have a power anti-inflammatory effect which is discussed later.

References
 1. Boulter, P. S., *Brit. J. Surg.* (1961), **49**, 17.
 2. Scott, M. E., and Orr., R., *Lancet* (1969), **i**, 1065–1067.
 3. Wright, N., and Syme, C. W., *Brit. Med. J.* (1969), **3**, 596.
 4. Rees, H. A., Muir, A. L., Macdonald, H. R., Lawrie, D. M., Burton, J. L., and Donald, K. W., *ibid.* (1967), **ii**, 863–866.
 5. Wijnja, L., Snijder, J. A. M., and Nieweg, H. O., *Lancet* (1966), **ii**, 768.
 6. Bell, D., Kerr, D. N. S., Swinney, J. and Yeates, W. K., *Brit. med. J.* (1969), **3**, 378–382.
 7. Editorial, *Lancet* (1969), **ii**, 1233.
 8. Aggeler, P. M., O'Reilly, R. A., Leong, L., and Kowitz, P. E., *New Eng. J. Med.* (1967), **276**, 9.
 9. Hart, F. D., and Boardman, P. L., *Brit. Med. J.* (1965), **ii**, 1281.
10. P. Hume-Kendall (Editor), *Fenamates in Medicine.* Suppl. to *Annals o, Physical Medicine* (1967).

This chapter was written by Dr W. G. Reeves (Dept of Clinical Pharmacology, Guys Hospital Medical School) and edited by Professor J. R. Trounce.

Category 4
Psychotropic Drugs

ANTIDEPRESSANTS

These drugs fall into two groups, namely the tricyclic compounds and monoamine oxidase inhibitors.* The former are discussed first.

Imipramine

Pharmacological action [1-2-3]. After absorption imipramine enters rapidly into the tissues from the blood stream. The highest concentration is in the brain and kidney, lowest in the liver except in overdosage. Its action is by inhibiting the uptake of noradrenaline and probably 5 hydroxy-tryptamine from synaptic clefts between cells of the CNS. Small quantities of the drug are excreted unchanged by the kidneys, whilst the major portion is metabolised within the body by de-methylation, hydroxylation and N-oxydation. Imipramine has anti-cholinergic and anti-histamine effects with weaker anti-emetic and hypothermic actions.

Therapeutic use [4-5]. Imipramine is used in endogenous and involutional depression with a consequent reduction in the number of electro-convulsive therapies required in severe forms. It is also used in the treatment of reactive depression and depression associated with schizophrenia and treatment of nocturnal enuresis. Oral starting dose for depression is 75 mg daily in divided doses, increasing gradually to 150-200 mg a day. There is minimal therapeutic effect for 14 days and it is not complete until six weeks; treatment is continued for four to six months when the drug should be gradually withdrawn. It may be given intramuscularly - 100 mg daily.

Contraindications and side effects. Use with caution in elderly people.
Imipramine is contraindicated in glaucoma and urinary retention. Side effects include dryness of the mouth, tachycardia, postural hypotension, constipation, difficulties in micturition, insomnia, drowsiness and tremor. Some patients complain of increased sweating and there

* Henceforth abbreviation M.A.O. will be used.

may be extrapyramidal symptoms with very large dosage and epilepsy in susceptible patients. Mild skin sensitivity to light, cholestatic jaundice and a few cases of agranulocytosis have been reported.

Desipiramine [6]

Trimipramine [7]

Opipramol

These three drugs resemble imipramine in most respects and should be given in similar dosage, except opipramol which is given in doses of 150–300 mg daily. Desipramine, the demethylated form, acts more rapidly but is less effective, and has less marked side effects. Trimipramine is as effective as imipramine. It produces greater drowsiness but is less hypotensive.

Opipramol an iminostilbene derivative with a piperazine side chain is more sedative but less efficacious than imipramine.

Amitriptyline [8]

Pharmacological action. A dibenzocycloheptene derivative similar to imipramine but with greater antihistaminic, anticholinergic and sedative effects.

Therapeutic use. Amitriptyline is useful in all forms of depression either alone or as an adjunct to ECT and particularly in agitated, elderly patients. The oral daily starting dose is 75–125 mg, part e.g. 50 mg may be given at night to assist sleep and reduce autonomic side effects during the day. The onset of action is in seven to ten days – its sedative action much sooner. Also intramuscularly 10–30 mg t.d.s.

Amitriptyline in tablets or syrup may be given to children in the treatment of nocturnal enuresis, usual starting dose being 25 mg at night.

Contraindications and side effects. As for imipramine but with greater autonomic manifestations. Drowsiness may be marked initially.

Nortripytline

Similar to amitriptyline but is more potent. Daily dosage of 30–100 mg, greater part of dose may be given at night to take advantage of sedative effects.

Protriptyline

This drug has stimulant properties and should be given with caution, ·average daily dose 15–60 mg. It may be given as a single dose in the morning followed by amitriptyline for the remainder of the day and at night.

Iprindole [9]

Pharmacological action. Similar to imipramine but minimal autonomic effects and less sedative than amitriptyline; excretion in faeces and urine.

Therapeutic action. All forms of depression, action is rapid and side effects are few. Oral dose: 30–60 mg t.d.s.

Contraindications and side effects. Care with MAO inhibitors.

Overdosage of tricyclic compounds. Caution is required in the use of these drugs in the elderly due to hypotensive side effects. Coma, respiratory depression, choreiform movements, convulsions, anomalies of cardiac conduction and hyperpyrexia may occur with toxic levels. Suicide is possible with as little as 4 g. of imipramine.

MONOAMINE OXIDASE INHIBITORS
HYDRAZINE DERIVATIVES

Iproniazid

Pharmacological action [10]. Absorbed from the gastrointestinal tract into the bloodstream and distributed to the tissues before reaching a high level in the brain, where it inhibits the oxidation of mono-amines. This action takes place in all areas of the brain with the probable exception of the corpus striatum. Within the cell action takes place at the level of the catecholamine storage vesicles.

Therapeutic use. Mainly in reactive depression and phobic anxiety states with a depressive element. A further use is in the treatment of ejaculatio praecox. Oral dosage of 50–150 mg a day, the greater part of the drug given in the morning and the rest at noon to prevent interference with sleep. Clinical response usually takes place within 5 days, but may take up to 3 weeks.

Contraindications and side effects. The most serious side effect of this drug is hepatocellular jaundice, which has an appreciable mortality and is the reason for it being withdrawn in the USA.

Isocarboxazide

Pharmacological action. Similar to iproniazid, metabolism is chiefly by hydrolysis to benzylhydrazine and a carboxylic compound; large quantities of hippuric acid reaching the urine.

Therapeutic use [11, 12]. The indications are similar to iproniazid but this drug, although more potent, is less effective clinically. Oral dose: 10–30 mg a day given early as above. It has a latent clinical response similar to iproniazid.

Contraindications and side effects. See below. Much reduced hepatotoxic effect as compared with iproniazid.

Nialamide

Pharmacological action. Similar to isocarboxazidazide but at least half the drug is excreted unchanged in the urine within 24 hours.

Therapeutic use. Similar indications to isocarboxazide but less efficacious. Oral dose: 75–150 mg a day given early as above with similar latent clinical response.

Contraindications and side effects (see below). Side effects are generally reduced with this drug but it is more hepatotoxic than isocarboxazide and should be given with care to agitated patients.

Phenelzine

Pharmacological action. Similar to iproniazid but with more activity in the brain and less in the liver.

Therapeutic use. Its marked sedative effect makes it particularly useful in reactive depression and phobic states with prominent anxiety. Oral dose: 45–90 mg a day given early and with similar latent clinical response as above.

Contraindications and side effects (see below). Reduced in comparison with other MAO inhibitors.

Mebanazine

Pharmacological action. Similar to phenelzine.

Therapeutic use. Similar to phenelzine. Oral dose 5–20 mg a day given early and with latent clinical response as above.

Contraindications and side effects (see below). Unsuitable with past history of liver disease or with impairment of hepatic or renal function.

Contraindications and side effects of MAO inhibitors.

MAO inhibitors potentiate the action of the following drugs: sympathomimetic agents such as adrenaline, ephedrine and amphetamine derivatives; morphine, pethedine and cocaine; guanethidine, reserpine and other hypotensive drugs; antiparkinsonian agents and barbiturates.

Preferably these agents should not be given for at least a fortnight after cessation of medication with MAO drugs. Great care should be taken in prescribing in combination with tricyclic antidepressants.

The oxidative deamination of tyramine which takes place in the walls of the gastrointestinal tract is blocked by MAO inhibitors. The following foodstuffs and drinks are contraindicated due to their large content of tyramine; cheese, broad beans, bananas, pickled herrings, certain protein and yeast extracts such as Bovril and Marmite; alcohol, including beer and certain wines such as Chianti.

Autonomic side effects include orthostatic hypotension; blurring of vision, dry mouth, warmer extremities with reduced sweating; constipation, micturition difficulties and impotence. Headaches, exacerbations of migraine and ankle oedema are met with. In the CNS drowsiness tremors and muscle jerks occur, as do manic states, toxic psychosis and exacerbation of schizophrenic symptoms.

Hepatocellular jaundice is seen in this group but to a variable extent as mentioned above.

Retrobulbar neuritis which usually resolves when the drug is discontinued; allergic skin reactions and exacerbations of eczema and asthma have been reported.

NON-HYDRAZINE DERIVATIVES

Tranylcypromine

Pharmacological action. Absorption and distribution are similar to preceding MAO inhibitors. Action in the brain resembles iproniazid, with the addition of amphetamine-like effects, which are sympathomimetic and stimulant to the ascending reticular formation. Metabolism is in part to hippuric acid; with other moieties entering the urine, and a small quantity of the drug is passed unchanged.

Therapeutic use [13]. Tranylcypromine is most effective in reactive and mixed depression where tiredness and lack of energy are prominent; it is contraindicated with marked tension and agitation. Oral dose: 20 mg a day in two doses before noon. Clinical response is faster than with hydrazine derivatives, but special precautions are required due to side effects.

Contraindications and side effects. Tranylcypromine can cause a gross hypertensive reaction with resultant transient hemiparesis or a subarachnoid haemorrhage. Habituation and true addiction occur. It is otherwise similar in side effects to hydrazine derivatives (see above).

Pargyline

This drug has MAO inhibitor properties, weak antidepressant action and is used for its hypotensive properties.

Overdosage of MAO inhibitors. Chief signs are marked drowsiness, depressed respiration, hypotonicity, fluctuations in blood pressure; and in presence of pressor agents headache, excitement, hallucinations, hypertension subarachnoid haemorrhage and coma.

Suicide is possible with less than 2 g.

Depression in Children [14].

Tricyclic compounds and less toxic MAO inhibitors may be used for treatment of anxiety and repression in older children and adolescents, in suitably adjusted doses.

LITHIUM

Lithium carbonate

Pharmacological action [15]. Lithium is widely distributed throughout the tissues following absorption from the gastrointestinal tract. Depressant action in the CNS probably depends upon the inhibition of enzymes and displacement of sodium. Excretion is chiefly in the urine.

Therapeutic use [16]. Lithium is claimed to be effective in mania, hypomania and for stabilisation of mood in manic depressive illness. In oral dosage the aim is to gain a serum level which lies between 0·8 and 1·5 mEq/1. Over 2·0 mEq/1 produces toxic signs. Weekly blood tests are therefore required over first two months. Starting dose with mania is 1–2 g. a day and maintenance of 0·5–0·75 g. a day with omission of the drug one day a week to minimise accumulation. It should not be combined with chlorpromazine as this increases the excretion of lithium.

Contraindications and side effects. Lithium is contraindicated in patients with heart failure, renal failure, Addison's disease or any tendency to electrolyte imbalance. Toxic signs include tremor, nausea, vomiting and diarrhoea, giddiness, ataxia, thirst, polyuria and drowsiness and coma. The drug should be withdrawn temporarily and serum level estimated at first signs of toxicity.

MAJOR TRANQUILLIZERS

1. PHENOTHIAZINES

Chlorpromazine

Pharmacological action [17]. Chlorpromazine is rapidly absorbed from the duodenum into the portal vein and thus to the liver where it is excreted via the bile and passed back to the gut for reabsorption. This cyclic process may be repeated and accounts for early conjugation observed after oral administration. Peak serum levels are usually obtained in thirty minutes and within the CNS in an hour: with highest concentrations appearing in mid-brain, medulla and pons. Parenteral administration has earlier peak levels and largely by-passes the enterohepatic route. Chlorpromazine depresses the brain stem reticular formation, its probable site of action being at the outer cell membrane with inhibition of amine transport. The drug is metabolised in the liver by demethylation, N-oxidation, sulphoxidation and hydroxylation. The latter is the chief route in formation of phenolic derivatives which conjugate with glucuronic acid. Glucuronides may be found in the urine, which is the main route of excretion, for up to thirty weeks after medication. The remainder of the metabolites are excreted in the faeces, 1 per cent being excreted in the urine as unchanged drug.

Therapeutic use [18, 19]. Chlorpromazine is used in psychotic illness; schizophrenia, states of mania and hypomania, acute and chronic brain syndromes, psychoneuroses, states of agitation, restlessness, excitement and acute anxiety. Also in personality disorders with tension, and with aggressive and destructive outbursts; in delirium tremens and withdrawal syndromes. In the treatment of acute schizophrenia there is argument as to whether chlorpromazine is antipsychotic or merely tranquillizing in action. In chronic schizophrenia it is valuable in controlling symptomatic exacerbations but is not thought to be useful on a long term basis with inactive and anergic patients. Oral dosage as sugar-coated tablets or syrup ranges from 65–600 mg a day although doses as high as 3,000 mg a day, in divided doses may be given for short periods. Dosage is highly individual and is not related to habitus or severity of symptoms but to metabolism. Oral administration is preferred but intramuscular injections in the range of 100 mg may be given to uncooperative patients, with due attention to physique, physical illness, prior medication and known sensitivity to this drug. Chlorpromazine injections may be painful.

Contraindications and side effects [20]. Chlorpromazine should be avoided in patients with a past history of jaundice and in those with glaucoma or prostatic hypertrophy. Side effects include initial drowsiness, and extrapyramidal symptoms in the elderly and with large dosage; these include weakness, tremor, rigidity, ataxia, loss of facial expression, excess salivation, restlessness and shuffling. Extreme dystonic reaction with gross bodily and facial contortions, protrusion of the tongue and oculogyric crises may occur. Autonomic effects include dryness of the mouth, nasal congestion, blurring of vision, urinary retention, constipation, tachycardia, ECG abnormalities and postural hypotension, especially in the elderly. Some cases of inhibition of ejaculation and paralytic ileus have been reported. Many patients gain weight, there may be disorders of menstruation, breast enlargement and lactation. With prolonged therapy the skin may become photosensitive and appears greyish from melanin deposition. Maculo-papular rashes occur and contact dermatitis is common in nursing staff. High dosage of over 500 mg a day may result in a pigmented retinopathy. Some patients develop an acute intrahepatic cholestatic jaundice which usually clears up when the drug is stopped. It very rarely progresses to cirrhosis. Blood dyscrasias, leucopaenia, granulocytopenia and agranulocytosis are rare but acute complications with high mortality rates; usually heralded by sore throat, malaise and fever. Myasthenia gravis may be precipitated or exacerbated.

Promazine

Pharmacological action. Similar to chlorpromazine; the chlorine atom of the phenothiazine nucleus is in this agent, replaced by hydrogen.

Therapeutic use [21]. As for chlorpromazine and in similar dose but less hepatotoxic and suitable for less acute cases.

Contraindications and side effects. As for chlorpromazine but greater tendency to agranulocytosis, and convulsions with large dosage and in patients with a past history of epilepsy.

Trifluopromazine

Pharmacological action. Similar to promazine but the carbon trifluoride radical reduces the tendency to fits.

Therapeutic use [21]. Oral dose: 50–300 mg t.d.s.

Methotrimeprazine

Pharmacological action. Thought to have analgesic effect and indicated in alcoholic withdrawal, depressive agitation and confusional states.

Therapeutic use. Oral dose: 5–50 mg t.d.s.

PIPERAZINE SIDE CHAIN COMPOUNDS

Trifluoperazine

Pharmacological action. Analagous to chlorpromazine, but substitution of piperazine side chain increases potency and carbon trifluoride radical reduces epileptogenic action.

Therapeutic use [21]. Chiefly in withdrawn, resistant cases of schizo-phrenia and especially with paranoid delusions; also in cases of chlor-promazine liver damage. Oral dose: 2–10 mg t.d.s.

Contraindications and side effects. Extrapyramidal effects may be marked and dystonic reactions common.

Perphenazine

Pharmacological action. Similar to chlorpromazine, whose chlorine atom it retains but perphenazine is more potent.

Therapeutic action [21]. Acutely disturbed patients. Oral dose: 2–24 mg t.d.s.

Contraindications and side effects. As for chlorpromazine.

Pericyazine

Pharmacological action. Analogous to chlorpromazine but more potent with substituted cyanide radical.

Therapeutic use. Thought to be useful in adolescent behaviour dis-orders and psychotic states. Oral dose: 5–50 mg t.d.s. Well tolerated intramuscularly, 10–20 mg dose.

Fluphenazine [21]

Replacement of the methyl group with an alcohol greatly strengthens its action. As effective clinically as chlorpromazine in schizophrenia. Useful in unreliable patients in form of depot injection 12·5–25 mg (fluphenazine enanthate) which lasts 2–4 weeks. Oral dose: 1–100 mg t.d.s.

Extra-pyramidal manifestations may be marked and severe de-pressive mood changes following depot injections have been reported.

Thiopropazate

The retained chlorine atom, provides little advantage over chlorpro-mazine except in treatment of Huntington's Chorea. Side effects often troublesome. Oral dose: 5–150 mg t.d.s.

PIPERIDINE SIDE CHAIN

Thioridazine [21]

Pharmacological action. Strongest acting member of this group and as effective as chlorpromazine but less extra-pyramidal manifestations and reduced photosensitivity.

Therapeutic use. Similar to chlorpromazine.

Useful in ejaculatio praecox; oral dose: 50–100 mg t.d.s.

Contraindications and side effects. Large dosage may produce pigmented retinopathy.

Overdose of Phenothiazine Group. Hypotension which may go on to circulatory collapse; hypothermia, dystonic reaction, oculogyric crises, convulsions and coma are also seen.

BUTYROPHENONES

Haloperidol

Pharmacological action. Related chemically to pethidine but with properties similar to phenothiazines.

Therapeutic use [22]. Haloperidol is indicated in psychotic states of mania, excitement and acute confusion. It is also used for habit spasm and tics, especially 'Giles de la Tourette' syndrome. The oral dosage is 3–10 mg a day in two to three divided doses; in uncooperative patients it can be given by intramuscular injection, 5–10 mg stat. and up to 15–45 mg total dose in a day.

Contraindications and side effects [23]. Extra-pyramidal symptoms can be troublesome and haloperidol should be given with care in the elderly and those affected by Parkinson's disease. It is usually combined with an anti-parkinsonian drug (see above). Its contraindications are glaucoma and urinary retention. Depression, loss of appetite and a symptomatic triad of sweating dehydration and hyperthermia have been described.

Triperidol

Pharmacological action. Similar to haloperidol.

Therapeutic action. This drug is more potent; oral dosage ranging from 1–3 mg a day.

Contraindications and side effects. Similar to those of haloperidol, but with greater extra-pyramidal effects.

TRICYCLIC COMPOUNDS RESEMBLING PHENOZIATHINES

Chlorprothixene

Pharmacological action. Similar to chlorpromazine with less extra-pyramidal effects, but greater anticholinergic symptoms.

Therapeutic use. Similar to chlorpromazine and particularly indicated in psychomotor agitation. Daily oral dose: 30–150 mg.

Clopenthixol

Pharmacological action. Similar to chlorpromazine but with stronger extra-pyramidal effects than chlorprothizene.

Therapeutic use. Anxiety associated with obsessional states and depression. Oral dose: 10–30 mg a day.

Contraindications and side effects. Less but in general similar to phenothiazines.

Oxypertine

This drug is an indol derivative with a piperazine side chain.

Therapeutic use. In schizophrenia, especially in withdrawn or apathetic patients. Oral dose 80–120 mg a day.

Contraindications and side effects. This drug produces extra-pyramidal manifestations.

Treatment of drug induced extra-pyramidal effects. These can be controlled with orphenadrine and benztropine (see above).

MINOR TRANQUILLIZERS

These drugs have sedative, hypnotic and relaxant properties.

1. BENZODIAZEPINES

Chlordiazepoxide [24]

Pharmacological action. Following absorption from the gastrointestinal tract this drug is widely distributed via the blood stream to all tissues. It acts as a depressant in the brain probably on the limbic system and has anticonvulsant and muscle relaxant properties. Metabolism is by hydroxylation and splitting which is followed by excretion, primarily in the urine and secondarily in the faeces.

Therapeutic use. Chlordiazepoxide relieves tension and anxiety, and its anticonvulsant properties indicate its use in the treatment of anxiety in epileptics. It is also used to alleviate symptoms of alcohol and drug-withdrawal syndromes.

Anxiety is a frequent presenting symptom of depression and may mask the underlying illness. Chlordiazepoxide is not an antidepressant and should be used in conjunction with antidepressant drugs when a depressive element is present.

Chlordiazepoxide may be used in the treatment of anxiety in children, also in conjunction with antidepressants in depression; and to promote relaxation leading to sleep.

Oral dosage is usually 10 mg t.d.s. with a daily range of 15–45 mg. Older patients may require smaller doses to avoid sleepiness and dosage must be suitably adjusted in children. It may be given as a hypnotic at night.

Contraindications and side effects. Drug dependence is possible but rare with chlordiazepoxide and withdrawal may produce convulsions. Confusion especially in the elderly, ataxia, pruritus, hypotension, loss of libido and excitement may occur. The appetite may be stimulated with consequent weight gain. There is potentiation of alcohol and barbiturates but suicide with this drug has not been reported.

Diazepam [24]

Pharmacological action. Similar to chlordiazepoxide but with stronger anticonvulsant and muscle relaxant properties.

Therapeutic use. Similar to chlordiazepoxide but more potent and particularly indicated in patients with marked tension producing muscle pains and headaches. Its stronger anticonvulsant properties make it useful in the treatment of drug withdrawal and it may be given intravenously in status epilepticus. Usual oral dose: 2–10 mg t.d.s.

Contraindications and side effects. Similar to chlordiazepoxide.

Oxazepam

Similar to chlordiazepoxide and most useful in the treatment of anxiety expressed as gastrointestinal, respiratory or cardiovascular symptoms. Sedative effects are said to be reduced. Oral dose: 15–30 mg t.d.s.

Nitrazepam

Pharmacological action. Similar to chlordiazepoxide but is said to have a selective depressant action on the limbic system and little effect upon the cerebral cortex and reticular formation.

Therapeutic use. Chiefly as a hypnotic but may be used as a sedative. Oral dosage: 5–10 mg at night or t.d.s.

2. SUBSTITUTED DIOLS

Meprobamate

Pharmacological action [24]. Meprobamate is rapidly absorbed from the gastrointestinal tract with distribution via the blood stream, initially to the visceral organs, peak levels being reached in about two hours in the CNS. It acts as a depressant in the brain on the limbic system and thalamus. It is largely metabolised within 24 hours by hydroxylation and conjugation of the drug with glucuronic acid followed by urinary excretion.

Therapeutic use [25]. In the management of mild anxiety state and tension but is unsuitable for severe anxiety. Its efficacy is open to some doubt. The oral dose is 800–1,600 mg a day and usually 400 mg t.d.s.

Contraindications and side effects. Meprobamate should not be used where there is a risk of drug dependence. A withdrawal syndrome is seen after prolonged medication consisting of restlessness, tremors, and ataxia with the possibility of convulsions and delirium. A commoner side effect is drowsiness, but sensitivity reactions occur with rash, pyrexia and fever. More rarely gastro-intestinal upsets, excitement, blood dyscrasias and paralysis of the extra-ocular muscles are seen.

The following drugs resemble meprobamate and are said to have sedative and relaxant properties:

Drug	Dose
1. Tybamate	350 mg t.d.s.
2. Phenaglycodol	200 mg q.d.s.
3. Oxanamide	400 mg t.d.s.
4. Emylclamate	200 mg t.d.s.
5. Mephenesin	500 mg t.d.s.
6. Carisoprodol	350 mg t.d.s.
7. Styramate	200 mg t.d.s.

3. THIAZOLE DERIVATIVES

Chlormethiazole

Pharmacological action. Not well understood after absorption from the gastrointestinal tract.

Therapeutic use. Claimed to be effective in the treatment of delirium tremens and confusional states. Dosage is 2 g. initially followed by 1 g. hourly until sleep ensues. Up to 8 g. may be given in 24 hours. Subsequent daily dosage should be gradually reduced, depending on the patient's state, and stopped in one to two weeks.

Contraindications and side effects. Sneezing and facial itching have been reported, hypotension and respiratory depression may occur.

4. DIPHENYLMETHANE DERIVATIVES

Azacyclonol
Pharmacological action. After absorption from the gastrointestinal tract azacyclonol is distributed primarily to brain. lungs and spleen. Site of action is uncertain but it is largely excreted in the urine within 24 hours.

Therapeutic use. Primarily for the treatment of hallucinations in schizophrenia but results have been disappointing. Average daily dose: 60–300 mg.

Contraindications and side effects. Rashes and hypotension may occur.

Benactyzine
Pharmacological action. Similar to azacyclonol.

Therapeutic use. Treatment of mild states of anxiety and depression. Oral dose: 3–6 mg daily.

Contraindications and side effects. Dryness of mouth, blurring of vision, poor concentration, feelings of mental retardation and increased anxiety have been reported.

Hydroxyzine
Pharmacological action. Similar to azacyclonol.

Therapeutic use. Mainly in states of anxiety and in psychogenic vomiting. Oral dose: 10–25 mg four times a day.

Contraindications and side effects. Headache, dry mouth and itching have been reported.

SEDATIVES

Barbiturates
These drugs are similar and will be described as a group.
Official Name

Phenobarbitone (Phenobarbital, *USA*)

Amylobarbitone (Amylobarbital, *USA*)

Pentobarbitone (Pentobarbital, *USA*)

Quinalbarbitone (Secobarbital, *USA*)
Pharmacological action. See above.

Therapeutic use. Barbiturates are used in minor states of anxiety, and the faster acting compounds in large dose in cases of acute disturbance. Individual response is wide and varied. They have been replaced in modern practice by the tranquillizers and particularly phenothiazines and butyrophenones in more acute states. However, intravenous barbiturates are still used as abreactive agents [27] often with methylamphetamine.

The following are the chief drugs in order of speed of sedative action:

Phenobarbitone, oral dose: 30 mg t.d.s.

Amylobarbitone, oral dose 15–45 mg t.d.s.

Amylobarbitone sodium, rapid action for acute anxiety, oral dose: 60–120 mg. In acutely disturbed patients by intramuscular or intravenous injection, 250–500 mg in 10 ml of water.

Pentobarbitone, oral dose: 100–200 mg.

Quinalbarbitone, oral dose: 100–200 mg.

Contraindications and side effects. Accumulation with subsequent depression may occur with phenobarbitone, and there are problems of tolerance and addiction for the group as a whole. Drowsiness, rash, and in the elderly, states of excitement and confusion may be troublesome.

PSYCHOTO-MIMETIC DRUGS [28]

Lysergide

Mescaline

Psylocybine

Piperidyl benzylate

Phencyclidine
Pharmacological action. These drugs are widely distributed following absorption, but there appears to be little correllation between brain concentrations and clinical effects. These may be divided into peripheral actions, including stimulation of muscle and vasoconstriction, and central

actions such as stimulation of sympathetic centres with tachycardia, hypertension, hyperglycaemia, pilo-erection and eye ball protrusion. Metabolism varies, with dephosphorylation, deamination and hydroxylation; piperidyl benzylate being rapidly excreted unchanged in the urine.

Therapeutic use. Their value is in dispute but lysergide, mescaline and psilocybine have been used to produce abreaction and as an aid to psychotherapy. The group as a whole have been used in the production of model psychoses for research purposes.

Contraindications and side effects. Schizophrenia, depression and obsessional states may be exacerbated and manic states precipitated in aggressive psychopaths.

References

 1. Domenjoz, R., and Theobald, W., *Archs. int. Pharmacodyn, Ther* (1959), **120**, 450.
 2. Holtz, P., and Westermann, E. (1965), *ibid.*, 1015.
 3. Pare, C. M. B., *Lancet* (1965), **i**, 923.
 4. Kuhn, R., *Amer. J. Psychiat.* (1958), **115**, 459.
 5. Medical Research Council, Report by Clinical Psychiatry Committee, *Brit. med. J.* (1965), **1**, 881.
 6. Dimascio, Heninger, G., and Klerman, G. L., *Psychopharmacologia* (1964), **5**, 361.
 7. Burns, B. H., *Brit. J. Psychiat.* (1965), **111**, 1155.
 8. Angst, J., *Psychopharmacologia* (1963), **4**, 389.
 9. Daneman, E. A., *Psychosomatics* (1967), **8**, 216.
10. Pscheidt, G. R., *Intern. Rev. Neurobiol* (1964), **7**, 191.
11. Crisp, A. H., Hays, P., and Carter, A., *Lancet* (1961), **i**, 17.
12. Richmond, P. W., and Roberts, A. H., *Brit. J. Psychiat.* (1964), **110**, 469.
13. Bartholomew, A. A., *Med. J. Aust.* (1962), **149**, 655.
14. Frommer, *Recent Developments in Affective Disorders* (1968), Headley Bros., Ashford.
15. Gershon, S., and Yuwiler, A., *J. Neuropsychiat.* (1960), 229.
16. Baastrup, P. C., and Schou, M., *Arch. gen. Psychiat.* (1967), **16**, 162.
17. Parkes, M. W., *in* Ellis, G. P., and West, G. B. (editors) *Progress in Medicinal Chemistry* (1961), **1**, Butterworths, London.
18. Freyhan, F. A., *Amer. J. Psychiat.* (1959), **115**, 577.
19. Malitz, S., *Ann. N.Y. Acad. Sci.* (1957), **66**, 717.
20. Hollister, L. E., *Clin. Pharmac. Ther.* (1964), **5**, 322.
21. Hanlon, T. E. *et al.*, *Psychopharmacologia* (1965), **7**, 89.
22. Trethowan, W. H., (editor) Proceedings of a Psychiatric Symposium on Haloperidol. *Clin. Trials J.* (1965), **2**, 133.

23. Gerle, B., *Acta Psychiat. scand.* (1964), **40**, 65.
24. Wittenborn, J. R., *The Clinical Psychopharmacology of Anxiety* (1966), Thomas Springfield, Illinois.
25. McNair, D. M. *et al.*, *Psychopharmacologia* (1965), **7**, 256.
26. Boyer, P. A., *Dis. Nerv. Syst.* (1966), **27**, 35.
27. Sargant, W., and Slater, E., *Physical Methods of Treatment in Psychiatry* (1963), Livingstone, Edinburgh.
28. Shepherd, M., Lader, M., and Rodnight, R., *Clinical Psychopharmacology* (1968), English Universities Press Limited, London.

This chapter was written by Dr J. B. Colville (Dept of Child and Adolescent Psychiatry, Guy's Hospital) and edited by Professor J. R. Trounce.

Category 5

Drugs Affecting the Autonomic Nervous System and Motor End-Plate

When considering the drugs which affect the autonomic nervous system and motor end-plate, it is useful to think in terms of four basic kinds of neuronal connection between the central nervous system and the end-organ. These are displayed diagramatically below. The chemi-

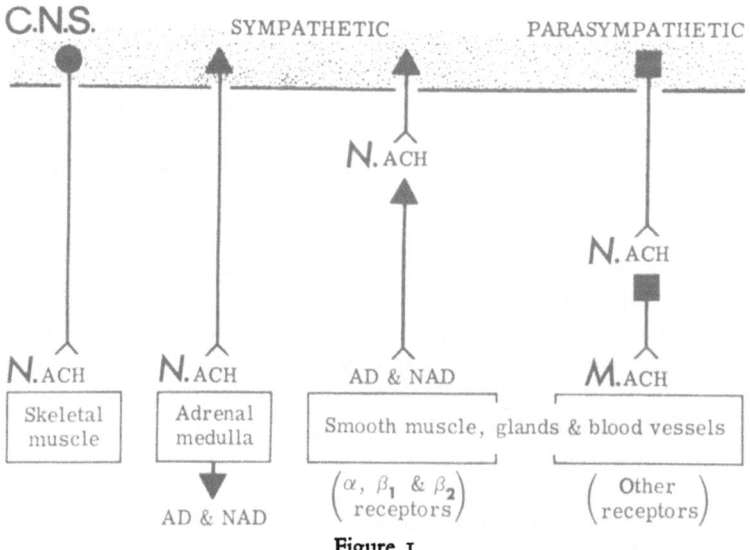

Figure 1.

N=nicotinic; M=muscarinic;   ACH=acetylcholine;
AD=adrenaline;   NAD=noradrenaline

cal transmitter at the first synapse in each case is acetylcholine. All these sites are 'nicotinic' as the effects of transmission can be mimicked by nicotine-like substances. The second synapse in the parasympathetic pathway is rather different and although dependent on acetylcholine as transmitter it is also stimulated by muscarine-like substances. In the

57

sympathetic pathway adrenaline and noradrenaline are the second synapse transmitter and the various end-organ receptors have been classified into α and β chiefly according to whether their effect is an excitatory or inhibitory one. This classification has proved useful but has required a little modification [1]. For further discussion of this subject see references [2] and [3].

Table 1

α Effects	β Effects
VASOCONSTRICTION particularly in skin and gut producing a rise in systolic and diastolic blood pressure with reflex showing of the heart. MYDRIASIS. ADRENERGIC SWEATING.	β_1 increased rate and force of contraction of the HEART. β_2 BRONCHODILATATION. VASODILATATION particularly of coronary vessels and vessels in skeletal muscle.

The drugs affecting the autonomic nervous system and motor end-plate will be discussed under the following headings:

1. Sympathomimetic Drugs.
2. Anti-adrenergic Drugs:
   (a) Post-ganglionic Neurone Blockers.
   (b) α and β Receptor Blockers
3. Parasympathomimetic Drugs.
4. Anti-cholinergic Drugs:
   (a) Ganglion Blockers
   (b) Neuromuscular Blockers
   (c) Drugs blocking muscarinic sites, i.e. Atropine and related drugs.

SYMPATHOMIMETIC DRUGS

Adrenaline (Epinephrine, USA)

Pharmacological action. Both α and β receptors are stimulated, its action resembling the activity of the sympathetic nervous system itself. Its α effects are to constrict blood vessels in skin and viscera, dilate the pupil and release glucose from the liver. The β effects are to increase the rate and force of contraction of the heart, dilate blood vessels in muscle and heart and dilate the bronchi. Like noradrenaline, it is inactive by mouth but has a rapid onset and short duration of action after subcutaneous injection.

Therapeutic uses. It is generally used as the acid tartrate or the hydrochloride. Dose: S.C. or I.M. 0·4–1 mg. It is often used locally in dilute solutions of varying strengths from 1 in 200,000 to 1 in 1,000, depending on the situation. It is not given intravenously. It is used to stop or reduce capillary bleeding both during and after surgery; to reduce nasal congestion; in combination with local anaesthetics (e.g. procaine) to prolong their action; to produce bronchodilatation in asthma; to counteract anaphylactic shock and other less serious allergic manifestations, e.g. urticaria, hay fever and angioneurotic oedema and to reverse heart block with syncope or even cardiac arrest. In the latter case it is often given as an intra-cardiac injection. It is also used as eye drops for retinoscopy and for open-angle (chronic simple) glaucoma in which situation it lowers the intra-ocular pressure. In narrow angle glaucoma it may increase the pressure.

Contraindications and side effects. It may produce feelings of anxiety, restlessness, palpitations, tachycardia, tremors, weakness, dizziness, headache and cold extremities. In excess it can cause cardiac arrhythmias and gangrene of extremities. It should not be used in very nervous or anxious patients or those with hypertension, ischaemic heart disease, hyperthyroidism, or in conjunction with trichlorethylene, halothane or cyclopropane. It is best avoided in patients who are receiving monoamine oxidase inhibitors.

Noradrenaline (Norepinephrine/Levarterenol, *USA*)

Pharmacological action. It has a predominant effect on α receptors causing vasoconstriction in muscle, skin and viscera, dilatation of the pupil, reduced muscular activity in the gastrointestinal and urinary tracts and glucose release from the liver. Both systolic and diastolic blood pressures rise and there is reflex slowing of the heart. It causes less cardiac stimulation than adrenaline.

Therapeutic uses. The acid tartrate is usually used, the dose being 2–20 μg/minute intravenously. Its chief use has been to treat hypotension in association with peripheral circulatory failure complicating myocardial infarction, the removal of phaeochromocytomas, the use of ganglion-blocking agents and many other conditions. The intense vasoconstriction usually restores the blood pressure but at the expense of adequate perfusion, especially of the kidneys. Latterly the trend has been to attach more significance to blood flow than pressure and to try and improve the former by using a combination of an α-adrenergic blocking agent and intravenous infusion of fluid [3]. Noradrenaline infusions should be stopped slowly as otherwise an abrupt fall in blood pressure may follow.

Contraindications and side effects. Gangrene of the extremities may follow prolonged infusions and severe phlebitis and necrosis around the site of injection has often been a sequel.

Isoprenaline (Isoproterenol, *USA*)

Pharmacological action. This is almost entirely on β receptors, producing a marked increase in the rate and force of contraction of the heart and relaxation of peripheral blood vessels, bronchi and most of the smooth muscle of the gut.

Therapeutic uses. It is usually given as the sulphate in a dose of 5–20 mg sublingually or by inhalation in an atomiser or as a pressurised aerosol. The hydrochloride is also used in a dose of 10 mg sublingually; or by inhalation or as a 0·02 per cent solution (1 in 5,000) subcutaneously. It can also be given I.M. or I.V. as an infusion. It is used widely in the control of bronchial asthma but has the disadvantage of stimulating the heart often to a considerably degree. The pharmacological separation of the β effects on heart and bronchial muscle [1] and the advent of drugs which have predominantly a β_2 effect, e.g. salbutamol, reduces this problem. It is only given by injection in the management of complete heart block and for long-term control it is best given as an oral sustained-release preparation, e.g. saventrine.

Contraindications and side effects. These include tachycardia, praecordial pain, hypotension, dizziness, headache, tremor and weakness. It should not be given in the presence of acute coronary insufficiency, heart failure and only with caution in hyperthyroidism.

Orciprenaline

Pharmacological action. An analogue of isoprenaline having similar β_1 and β_2 effects and which is fully active when swallowed.

Therapeutic uses. It is used almost entirely as a bronchodilator. Dose:

orally 10–20 mg; as a 5 per cent solution by inhalation or 0·5 mg S.C. or I.M.
Contraindications and side effects. As isoprenaline but usually less troublesome.

Salbutamol
Pharmacological action. A drug which stimulates β_2 receptors in bronchial muscle but which has little or no effect on β_1 receptors in the heart.
Therapeutic uses. This has considerable advantages over isoprenaline in the management of bronchial asthma as it does not have the risk of precipitating untoward cardiac effects, e.g. arrhythmias [4]. It is given as a pressurised aerosol discharging puffs of 100 μg. Dose 100–400 μg. It can also be used as tablets in a dose of 5 mg b.d. or t.d.s.
Contraindications and side effects. So far remarkably few side effects have been seen.

Ephedrine
Pharmacological action. This is similar to adrenaline as it has both α and β effects, although its effect is slower and more sustained. It acts partly on the receptor directly but also by releasing noradrenaline from stores at adrenergic nerve endings. It may also work partly by inhibiting amine-oxidase. It has a greater stimulating effect on the central nervous system in adults although children may be sedated. It is effective orally.
Therapeutic uses. Dose: 15–60 mg orally or subcutaneously as the hydrochloride or sulphate. It is also used as a 1 per cent spray. Its chief use is as a bronchodilator. It is sometimes used to increase conduction in complete heart block, to alleviate narcolepsy and cataplexy and to augment the effect of neostigmine in myasthenia. It is also useful in the management of enuresis.
Contraindications and side effects. Large doses may cause headache, nausea, vomiting, palpitations, difficulty in micturition, muscular weakness, tremors, anxiety, restlessness and insomnia. It should not be given to elderly men and those in whom prostatism is suspected. It should not be used in the presence of ischaemic heart disease, hypertension and thyrotoxicosis.

Amphetamine
Pharmacological action. A sympathomimetic drug with a marked stimulating effect on the central nervous system. It lessens fatigue, gives

a feeling of well-being and can easily produce a state of habituation or addiction, especially following indiscriminate use. It also suppresses appetite.

Therapeutic uses. Dose: orally 5–10 mg. It has been used in the management of narcolepsy and occasionally in epilepsy and parkinsonism. Other agents have now largely replaced it in all these situations in view of the very real danger of habituation. It should not be used as a tonic, to reduce appetite or to treat depression. It should not be given with MAO inhibitors.

Dexamphetamine
Pharmacological action and therapeutic uses. This has the same effects, uses and disadvantages as amphetamine.

Methylphenidate
Pharmacological action and uses. This has a similar action to amphetamine but is the recommended antidote for pentazocine (q.v.) overdosage as nalorphine is ineffective.

Hydroxyamphetamine
Pharmacological action and therapeutic uses. This has an effective vasopressor action without the central effects of amphetamine. It also has a direct stimulating action on the heart. It has been used to correct hypotension, bradycardia and as a nasal decongestant and mydriatic. Dose: orally 20–60 mg; I.M. 10–20 mg and I.V. 5–10 mg.

Methylamphetamine (Methamphetamine, *USA*)
Pharmacological action and therapeutic uses. These are the same as for amphetamine with the exception that I.M. or I.V. it is an effective α-stimulator and produces a vasopressor effect in a dose of 10–30 mg. Its central stimulant effects are marked even in small doses and this has led to its vogue as a drug of addiction.

Methoxyphenamine
Pharmacological action and therapeutic uses. This drug has little vasopressor activity but does dilate bronchi and is used in the control of asthma. Dose: orally 50–100 mg every 3 or 4 hours.

There are many other sympathomimetic drugs which have been used as vasopressor agents. These include:

Cyclopentamine/Mephentermine/Metaraminol/
Methoxamine/Phenylephrine/Phenylpropranolamine

Most of them are α stimulators although metaraminol has both α and β effects and mephentermine has almost entirely a β stimulating effect.

ANTI-ADRENERGIC DRUGS

α BLOCKING AGENTS

Phentolamine

Pharmacological action. This is similar to tolazoline (q.v.) although it is rather more potent and has a shorter duration of action. It acts by competing with α-stimulating agents for the α receptor and its effects can be reversed by giving large amounts of these drugs. It is not reliably effective when given orally.

Therapeutic uses. Dose: orally 40–100 mg 4 to 6-hourly as the hydrochloride or I.V. 5–10 mg as the mesylate. The latter is used chiefly in the diagnosis of phaeochromocytoma. In this situation a fall in blood pressure of at least 35/25 mm Hg should occur within 2 minutes of giving 5 mg I.V. Orally, phentolamine has been given for the control of hypertension in phaeochromocytoma prior to surgery.

Parenterally it can also be used as an antidote to adrenaline or noradrenaline.

Contraindications and side effects. Orally it may cause nausea, vomiting, diarrhoea and gastrointestinal disturbances. Less often tachycardia, praecordial pain and postural hypotension are troublesome.

Phenoxybenzamine

Pharmacological action. A powerful α-blocker which acts for longer than phentolamine; its effect lasting for several days. It probably alters the receptor in some way rather than acting by competition and its effects cannot be reversed by noradrenaline. The maximum effect of an I.V. injection may take an hour to develop.

Therapeutic uses. Dose: orally 10–20 mg initially, subsequent doses to be determined according to the patient's response. It has been used for peripheral vascular disease but is not suitable for the control of hypertension, other than that due to phaeochromocytoma, because of side effects which usually develop with the dose levels required. Latterly it has been used in the management of peripheral circulatory failure in combination with the intravenous infusion of fluid and central venous pressure monitoring [5]. This is in preference to the previous vogue of giving α-stimulators, e.g. noradrenaline (norepinephrine) which produces marked vasoconstriction but at the cost of a severe reduction in flow and tissue perfusion. I.V. a total daily dose of 0·5–1 mg/kg body-weight is given in 250–500 ml normal saline or dextrose injection over a period of at least 1 hour.

Contraindications and side effects. It should not be given where a fall in blood pressure would be dangerous. A single large dose can cause postural hypotension lasting for 2 days or more. Other side effects include nasal congestion, dry mouth, pupillary constriction, drowsiness, fatigue and weakness. Anorexia, nausea, vomiting and other gastro-intestinal disturbances tend to occur more with oral therapy.

Thymoxamine

Pharmacological action. This is a potent and fairly specific α-blocking agent having a marked vasodilator effect. It produces its effect by a competitive and reversible blockade of the α-receptors.

Therapeutic uses. Dose: orally 5–10 mg 3 or 4 times daily; or 5–30 mg daily S.C. or I.M. or by slow I.V. injection. Its chief use is as a peripheral vasodilator.

Contraindications and side effects. These include nausea, diarrhoea, facial flushing, vertigo and headache, but are less severe than those seen with phentolamine.

Some phenothiazines, e.g. chlorpromazine hydrochloride, also have an α-blocking effect which is strong enough to cause hypotension. Some ergot alkaloids have α-blocking activity but this is usually masked by their powerful direct vasoconstrictor effect.

β-BLOCKING AGENTS

D.C.I. [Dichloroisoprenaline (*UK*), Dichloroisoproterenol (*USA*)] was the first drug of this class but in addition it had some of the sympathomimetic activity of isoprenaline and is not now used. Another drug pronethalol was withdrawn because it produced tumours in animals.

Propranolol

Pharmacological action. A powerful and fairly specific β-blocker which probably acts by competition with catecholamines for the β-receptors. This produces a reduction in the rate and force of contraction of the heart. It also has a quinidine-like and a local anaesthetic effect, reducing the rate of ectopic foci. Even in normal people it causes mild bronchial constriction which is much more marked in asthmatics.

Therapeutic uses. Its uses in the treatment of angina, cardiac arrhythmias and hypertension are discussed elsewhere. It is also used in the management of phaeochromocytoma in association with α-blocking agents which should usually precede its administration. For details see [6].

Several new β-blocking agents have recently been the subject of drug trials. These include practolol (I.C.I.50172), oxyprenol (trasicor) and alprenol. To date, practolol would appear to show some advantages and will be discussed here.

Practolol
A recently developed drug which seems to block β_1 receptors in the myocardium without blocking β_2 receptors in bronchi or peripheral vessels [7, 8]. It also differs from propranolol in that it has no quinidine-like or local anaesthetic effect but does have weak sympathomimetic activity [9].

Therapeutic Uses
It promises to be superior to propranolol in the treatment of angina pectoris and cardiac arrhythmias. It does not tend to induce bronchoconstriction or cardiac failure and is especially useful in the management of arrhythmias following myocardial infarction [10]. Dose I.V. 5–25 mg, orally 50 mg b.d. A maximum dose of 600 mg daily for control of arrhythmias and 1 g. daily for angina has been used.

Contraindications and side effects
Any degree of atrio-ventricular block in association with a slow heart-rate is taken as an absolute contraindication. Otherwise it seems to give rise to much fewer side-effects than propranolol.

PARASYMPATHOMIMETIC DRUGS

CHOLINE ESTERS

Methacholine
Pharmacological action. Like acetylcholine it stimulates the parasympathetic nervous system but has predominantly a muscarinic effect. It chiefly affects the cardiovascular system causing bradycardia and dilata-

tion of peripheral blood vessels. It increases salivation, sweating and bronchial secretion.

Therapeutic uses. Dose: orally 10–500 mg; S.C. 10–25 mg. It is not given intravenously. Methacholine bromide is sometimes used and has a similar action. Dose: orally 200–600 mg. Methacholine has been used to stop supraventricular tachycardias and to stimulate the bowel and bladder, although carbachol is probably better for the latter.

Contraindications and side effects. These include nausea, vomiting, flushing, increased salivation, involuntary defaecation, bradycardia, transient heart block, hypotension, dyspnoea and substernal discomfort. If given by injection it may give rise to a terrifying feeling of choking. It should not be given to patients with asthma, hypertension, ischaemic heart disease, Addison's disease or peptic ulceration. Serious reactions have resulted from the combined use of methacholine and neostigmine.

Carbachol

Pharmacological action. It has both muscarinic and nicotinic effects but chiefly affects the gastrointestinal tract.

Therapeutic uses. Dose: S.C. 0·25 mg repeated up to 2 or 3 times at 30-minute intervals. It is also used in a 0·8 per cent aqueous solution as eye drops. Its most frequent use is for post-operative intestinal atony and retention of urine. It has also been used for supraventricular tachycardias and is occasionally used as a miotic. Unwanted side effects can be reversed with atropine 0·6 mg S.C.

Contraindications and side effects. It may cause sweating, nausea, faintness, colic and diarrhoea. It should not be used in the presence of mechanical obstruction in the gastrointestinal or urinary tracts or after gastrointestinal anasomosis. It is less safe in the elderly.

Bethanechol

Pharmacological action. This is similar to methacholine but it is not destroyed by choline-esterase. It is less toxic and less active than methacholine.

Therapeutic use. Dose: orally 5–30 mg up to 3 times a day; S.C. 2·5–5 mg at no less than 4-hourly intervals. It is the best tolerated of these three drugs for the treatment of postoperative intestinal stasis (e.g. after vagotomy) and distension, and is also useful for postoperative urinary retention.

Contraindications and side effects. As carbachol but less troublesome.

CHOLINE-ESTERASE INHIBITORS

Physostigmine

Pharmacological action. It potentiates the action of acetylcholine by inhibiting choline-esterase. It thus produces muscarinic and nicotinic effects as well as acting on the central nervous system. It is particularly useful as a miotic acting within 10 minutes of local application, the effect lasting for about 12 hours.

Therapeutic uses. It is now only used as eye-drops. It is useful for the relief of glaucoma and to counteract the dilatation produced by atropine or cocaine. It is usually used as a 0·25 per cent solution, higher concentrations often causing irritation.

Neostigmine

Pharmacological action. This has a similar action to physostigmine although the nicotinic effects are more and the muscarinic effects less prominent. It is thus used chiefly for its effect on skeletal muscle.

Therapeutic uses. Preparations: N. bromide – orally, N. methylsulphate – by injection. It is still the mainstay of treatment for myasthenia gravis and is used in a dose of 15–30 mg orally three or four times daily. It can be given by I.M. or I.V. injection 1–2·5 mg several times daily up to a total of 3 mg/day. It has also been used as a diagnostic aid for myasthenia in a dose of 1–1·5 mg I.M. or I.V. Increase in muscular power with improvement in symptoms should be noticeable within 15 minutes. Neostigmine is also used as an antidote to the muscle relaxants tubocurarine and gallamine. 2·5–5 mg is given I.V. after 0·5–1 mg atropine I.V.

Contraindications and side effects. Toxic effects include restlessness, weakness, nausea, vomiting, diarrhoea and abdominal pain. Increased sweating, salivation and lachrymation occur, and if excessive doses are given generalised muscular twitching convulsions and collapse may ensue. The muscarinic effects can be controlled with atropine. Neostigmine should not be used in patients with asthma, ischaemic heart disease, parkinsonism, epilepsy, bradycardia, hypotension, and intestinal or urinary tract obstruction.

Pyridostigmine

Pharmacological action. Similar to neostigmine but with a quarter of the potency. It is slower in onset, acting within 30–45 minutes and lasting for 4–6 hours.

E

Therapeutic uses. It is used, often in association with neostigmine, for myasthenia gravis, in a dose of 60-240 mg orally and 1-5 mg S.C. or I.M.

Contraindications and side effects. As neostigmine.

Ambenonium

Pharmacological action and therapeutic uses. Similar to neostigmine but longer lasting. It is used for myasthenia gravis especially when neostigmine is poorly tolerated. Dose: 5-25 mg three or four times daily.

Contraindications and side effects. As neostigmine but less marked.

Benzypyrinium

Pharmacological action and therapeutic uses. Another very similar compound. Dose: 2 mg I.M.

Edrophonium

Pharmacological action. Similar to neostigmine but its effect on skeletal muscle is much more marked and most of its effect is probably due to a direct action on the muscle receptor rather than inhibition of cholineesterase. It has a rapid onset and short duration of action.

Therapeutic use. It is particularly useful in the diagnosis of myasthenia gravis. A test dose of 2 mg is given I.V. and if there has been no untoward effect after 30 seconds a further 8 mg is given. With myasthenia there is immediate improvement and increase in muscle power which disappears within 5 minutes. It is therefore not suitable for routine use. It is also suitable for deciding in a myasthenic patient between weakness due to too much or too little neostigmine.

Contraindications and side effects. As neostigmine but very short-lived.

Dyflos (DFP)

Pharmacological action. Causes prolonged inhibition of choline-esterase as do many of the organophosphates. Its effect may last for two weeks and thus it is not suitable for systemic use. Its action resembles neostigmine and physostigmine and its particular value is as a miotic.

Therapeutic use. Eye drops are made up as a 10 per cent solution in arachis oil. Dose: 1 drop t.d.s. It is used as a miotic for glaucoma.

Contraindications and side effects. Ocular pain often occurs initially and there may be a transient rise in intra-ocular pressure. After prolonged medication iris cysts may develop which usually regress after treatment has ceased. DFP can be absorbed through the skin, conjunctiva and respiratory and gastrointestinal tracts. Its vapour is very toxic and thus eye drops are made up in an oily substance. Systemic administration via one or more of these routes leads to ciliary and iris spasm, transient bronchial constriction, muscle fibrillation, salivation, diarrhoea, urinary retention, restlessness, headache, convulsions and collapse.

Most of these effects of poisoning can be controlled by I.M. or I.V. injections of 1–2 mg atropine sulphate. This may be repeated every 10–30 minutes until signs of atropinisation appear. 20 mg or more may be required. A specific choline-esterase reactivor, e.g. Pralidoxime (UK and USA) should be given (dose: 1–2 g. daily, I.M. or I.V.) and repeated as necessary. Artificial ventilation may be required.

Contraindications are as for neostigmine, with the additional exclusion that it should not be used for acute congestive (narrow angle) glaucoma as here it may cause a further rise in pressure; neither should it be used in the presence of retinal damage.

Ecothiopate
Pharmacological action and therapeutic uses. Very similar to dyflos. It is used as a miotic. It is usually used as an 0·25 per cent aqueous solution. Dose: from 1 drop alternate days to twice a day.

Contraindications and side effects. As dyflos.

PILOCARPINE

Pilocarpine
Pharmacological action. An alkaloid having the muscarinic effects of acetycholine with little of its nicotinic effects. It is used chiefly as a miotic and has about half the activity of physostigmine and acts for a shorter length of time. It has also been used to counteract the side effects of ganglion-blocking agents.

Therapeutic uses. As a miotic it is used as a 1 per cent solution; orally it is given in a dose of 2·5–12 mg.

Contraindications and side effects. Increased salivation, sweating and production of tears predominate. With excessive doses nausea, vomiting, diarrhoea, dyspnoea, confusion, tremor and convulsions may occur.

GANGLION-BLOCKING AGENTS

Hexamethonium/Mecamylamine/Pempidine/Pentolinium/ Trimetaphan

These are now chiefly used for the rapid control of an elevated blood pressure and are discussed in the section on HYPOTENSIVE DRUGS.

NEUROMUSCULAR BLOCKING AGENTS

DEPOLARISING AGENTS

Suxamethonium (Succinylcholine, USA)

Pharmacological action. This drug acts by depolarising voluntary muscle in a similar way to acetylcholine but as suxamethonium (succinylcholine) is destroyed less quickly the depolarisation temporarily persists. The onset of relaxation is preceded by a short period of contraction which causes pain if the patient is conscious, and probably causes the muscle pain which occurs for up to 3 days after its use. The effect of this drug is not reversed by cholinergic drugs. It is destroyed by plasma pseudo-cholinesterase.

Therapeutic uses. Dose: 30–50 mg I.V. It is used as a short-acting muscle relaxant in conjunction with major and minor surgical and manipulative procedures.

Contraindications and side effects. Prolonged apnoea will occur in those with a low or atypical plasma pseudo–cholinesterase. The former may occur with liver disease, severe anaemia, malnutrition or after treatment with anticholinesterases, e.g. neostigmine. The latter is an hereditary defect. A prolonged effect may also follow if streptomycin or neomycin is given soon after the administration of suxamethonium. Repeated doses can cause bradycardia and arrhythmias. Generalised muscle pain is a common after-effect and can be prevented by giving a small dose of a competitive blocking agent before the suxamethonium.

NON-DEPOLARISING AGENTS

Tubocurarine

Pharmacological action. This drug acts by competing with acetylcholine for the receptors on the motor end-plate. It does not cause depolarisation but prevents its occurrence due to acetylcholine. This causes a flaccid paralysis. It develops within a minute of I.V. injection and lasts for 20–45 minutes. Tubocurarine also has a ganglion-blocking effect and causes tissue histamine to be released. These effects explain the occasional occurrence of a fall in blood pressure and the development of bronchospasm.

The action of tubocurarine is reversed by anticholinesterase drugs, e.g. neostigmine methylsulphate 2·5–5 mg I.V. preceded by 0·5–1 mg atropine I.V. to prevent the parasympathetic effects of the neostigmine.

Therapeutic uses. Dose: initially 5 mg I.V. as a test dose followed in 5 minutes by 10–20 mg I.V. Additional dose of 2–4 mg can be given at 30 minute intervals up to a total dose of 45 mg.

Dimethyltubocurarine bromide, chloride or iodide can be used instead of tubocurarine chloride and these drugs are all roughly three times as potent requiring about a third of the above dose. This drug is used to produce muscular relaxation during surgery and is also used to control muscle spasm and convulsions in tetanus.

Contraindications and side effects. It is rarely toxic but may occasionally lower the blood pressure and cause bronchospasm. Administration of tubocurarine before or after the use of suxamethonium can cause a state of neostigmine-resistant curarisation. This will require continued ventilation but usually settles after a few hours. It tends to occur in patients who are dehydrated, hypokalaemic or otherwise metabolically disturbed. Tubocurarine should not be used in patients with myasthenia or those with respiratory, hepatic or renal disease. Patients with carcinomatous neuromyopathies often give abnormal and prolonged responses to muscle relaxants. Potentiation occurs with ether, chlorpromazine and some antibiotics (e.g. streptomycin, neomycin and polymyxin).

Gallamine

Pharmacological action. It is similar to tubocurarine but has little effect on autonomic ganglia. It does not produce histamine release and is less potent and shorter-acting. Relaxation starts within 2 minutes and lasts for about 20 minutes.

Therapeutic uses. Dose: 80–120 mg I.V. Up to half of the initial amount can be given as a second dose. It is used to obtain shorter periods of muscular relaxation during surgery and to minimise the convulsions of shock therapy. Premedication with atropine is necessary to prevent excessive salivation.

Contraindications and side effects. As tubocurarine. In addition it may produce allergic reactions in people sensitive to iodine and occasionally causes a tachycardia which persists for a while after the relaxant effect has disappeared.

ATROPINE AND RELATED DRUGS

Atropine (dl-Hyoscyamine)
Pharmacological action. Centrally it initially stimulates and later depresses the nervous system. It reduces tremor and muscular rigidity especially in people with parkinsonism and may help oculogyric crises although the mechanism is unknown. Peripherally it blocks the muscarinic effects of acetylcholine and thus antagonises all the effects of acetylcholine except for those at autonomic ganglia and the neuromuscular junction. It has an antispasmodic action on smooth muscle and decreases secretions. It depresses vagal activity causing slowing of the heart. It is also an antiemetic.

On the eye it has both a mydriatic and cycloplegic action and may cause a rise in intraocular pressure.

Therapeutic uses. Dose: 0·25–2 mg orally, S.C. or I.M. Its effect on the gut is utilised in the treatment of peptic ulceration and pylorospasm. In congenital hypertrophic pyloric stenosis it is usually given as atropine methonitrate (UK)/atropine methylnitrate (USA) in a dose of 2–6 ml of a 0·01 per cent aqueous solution half an hour before feeds. The methonitrate has less effect on the central nervous system and is less toxic to infants. It is also used to control bronchial asthma in a compound adrenaline and atropine spray or as the methonitrate alone in a pressurised aerosol. However atropine may make bronchial secretions extremely viscid and sympathomimetic agents are often preferred.

Atropine is often used for its effect on the heart, e.g. to prevent vagal syncope and to correct the bradycardia due to digitalis, opiates, choline esters, pilocarpine or anticholine esterases. It has also been used for partial heart block. It is used as a premedication in view of its ability to reduce secretions and protect the heart from vagal inhibition. It has been used in parkinsonism and will also reduce the sialorrhoea, but other atropine-like agents, e.g. benzhexol are probably more suitable.

Atropine has an antiemetic effect but other drugs, e.g. cyclizine, meclozine, etc. cause less side effects. As a mydriatic and cycloplegic it is used as 1 per cent eye drops. Dilatation occurs within 30 minutes and may last 2 weeks. For this reason homatropine is usually preferred.

Contraindications and side effects. These include dry mouth, thirst, dilatation of pupils with loss of accommodation and photophobia, flushing, difficulty with micturition and constipation. Toxic doses cause restlessness, excitement, confusion and hallucinations, tachycardia and hyperpyrexia. Later drowsiness, stupor and generalised central depression may occur. Side effects may even occur with eye drops. Atropine must not be used on patients with a narrow angle between the iris or cornea or those who have developed glaucoma. It should be used with care in those with prostatic enlargement, ischaemic heart disease or cardiac failure, and should not be used in paralytic ileus. The danger of hyperpyrexia should be considered in unduly hot weather or climates.

Hyoscine (scopolamine)

Pharmacological action. Similar to atropine although its effect on the central nervous system is between 3 and 10 times as potent. This is usually a depressant effect although excitement can occur especially in the elderly.

Mydriasis is quicker in onset and of shorter duration.

Therapeutic uses. Dose: as atropine. It has been used for acute mania, parkinsonism and as an hypnotic. It is also used as a premedication, usually in combination with an opiate, and as a mydriatic.

Contraindications and side effects. As atropine but it should be avoided in the elderly.

Hyoscine hydrobromide

Pharmacological action. Very similar actions and uses to hyoscine.

Therapeutic use. Dose: 0·3–0·6 mg S.C.

Hyoscine butylbromide

Pharmacological action. It is often ineffective orally but parenterally it is an effective smooth muscle relaxant and is used for this effect on the cardia, stomach, colon and biliary and renal tracts. It does not have much effect on gastric secretion and unlike hyoscine it also has a blocking action at ganglia. Dose: 20–40 mg S.C. or I.M.; 10–20 mg I.V.

Hyoscine methobromide (Methscopolamine bromide, USA)

Pharmacological action. A quarternary amine which thus lacks the central action of atropine and is a more selective inhibitor of gastric secretion. It is longer acting than hyoscine.

Therapeutic use. Dose: orally 2·5–5 mg 8-hourly; 0·25 to 1 mg S.C. or I.M. three or four times a day.

Homatropine hydrobromide

Pharmacological action. Similar to atropine but rather weaker. As a mydriatic its action is more rapid and less prolonged although it may last for 24 hours. The dilatation is easily reversed with physostigmine.- It is rarely used systemically although the methobromide has been used for its effect on the gastrointestinal tract.

Therapeutic use. Dose: 0·5–2 mg as a 1 or 2 per cent solution.

Cyclopentolate

Pharmacological action and uses. A mydriatic and cycloplegic agent quicker and shorter-acting than homatropine. Mydriasis develops within 10–20 minutes and cycloplegia soon after; the effect lasting for 6–12 hours. Dose: 1–2 drops of a 0·5 or 1 per cent solution. Its effect is best reversed by pilocarpine.

Lachesine

Pharmacological action and uses. A mydriatic and cycloplegic agent having a slower onset of action which is less prolonged than atropine, achieving a maximum at 1 hour and disappearing within 6 hours. It does not cause conjunctival irritation and is a useful alternative for those patients who show a sensitivity to substances of the atropine group. Usual dose is 2 drops of a 1 per cent solution.

Propantheline

Pharmacological action. It is one of many synthetic anticholine drugs and has a marked peripheral atropine-like effect with little effect on the CNS. It is also a weak ganglion-blocker and at very high doses has a curare-like effect on the neuromuscular junction.

Therapeutic uses. Dose: 15–30 mg orally, I.M. or I.V. Its more frequent use is to reduce gastric intestinal secretion and motility. It is an effective antispasmodic and may be given with an opiate for visceral colic to reduce the stimulating effect of the former on smooth muscle.

Contraindications and side effects. As for atropine with the additional hazard that in toxic doses paralysis of voluntary muscle may occur.

There are many more anticholinergic agents which have been developed for systemic use, chiefly for their effects in reducing spasm, motility and secretion in the gastrointestinal tract. Four further drugs will be mentioned by name, although they differ little from propantheline in their actions, uses and side effects.

Poldine

Pharmacological action and uses. This is a potent inhibitor of gastric secretion with a prolonged action. Dose: 2–4 mg orally, 6-hourly, but this often requires adjustment as atropine-like side effects are common at the higher dose levels.

Dicyclomine

Pharmacological action and uses. It is an antispasmodic similar to but weaker than atropine. It has also a mild local anaesthetic action. Dose: 10–20 mg orally, three or four times daily.

Tricyclamol

Pharmacological action and uses. Similar to atropine; it also has ganglion blocking activity in large doses. Dose: 50–100 mg orally four- or six-hourly before meals.

Isopropamide

Pharmacological action and uses. Similar to tricyclamol except that it has a more prolonged action. Dose: orally 5 mg 8–12-hourly.

References

1. Lands, A. M., Arnold, A., McAuliff, J. P., Luduena, F. P., and Brown, T. G., *Nature* (1967), (London), **214**, 597–8.
2. Burn, J. H., and Dornhorst, A. C., *In Recent Advances in Pharmacology* (1968), J. & A. Churchill, London. Edited by Robson, J. M., and Stacey, R. S., 4th Edition.
3. Turner, P., *In Fifth Symposium on Advanced Medicine* (1969), Edited by Roger Williams, Pitman Medical.
4. Palmer, K. N. V., and Diament, M. L., *Brit. med. J.* (1969), **1**, 31–32.
5. Riordan, J. F., and Walters, G., *ibid.*, 155–158.
6. Ross, E. J., Prichard, B. N. C., Kaufman, L., Robertson, A. I. G., and Harries, B. J., *ibid.* (1967), **1**, 191.
7. Turner, P., *Clinical Aspects of Autonomic Pharmacology* (1969), Heinemann.
8. Palmer, K. N. V., Legge, J. S., Hamilton, W. F. D., and Diament, M. L., *Lancet* (1969), **ii**, 1092.
9. Wilson, A. G., Brooke, O. G., Lloyd, H. J., and Robinson, B. F., *Brit. med. J.* (1969), **4**, 399.
10. Jewitt, D. E., Mercer, C. J., and Shillingford, J. P., *Lancet* (1969), **ii**, 227.

This Chapter was written by Dr W. G. Reeves (Department of Clinical Pharmacology, Guy's Hospital Medical School) and edited by Professor J. R. Trounce.

Category 6

Drugs Used in Cardiac Disease

Digoxin

Pharmacological action. Digoxin is a pure glycoside obtained from the leaves of Digitalis lanata.

The action of the digitalis glycosides at the cellular level is uncertain, but it is possible that they affect the movement of ions across the cell membrane in such a way as to reduce the sodium and potassium gradients, whilst conserving calcium within the cell. The result of the former is to lead to an increased ease of depolarisation of the cell membrane – this could explain the toxic effects on the heart – and of the latter is to improve the contractility of the muscle fibre. In addition to these direct cellular actions the cardiac glycosides are known to increase vagal control of the heart.

The effects of digitalis glycosides are most readily seen in patients with cardiac failure and tachycardia, in whom they lower the venous pressure and slow the heart rate. Part of this slowing can be blocked by atropine but part is due to a direct action on the SA node. A greater slowing effect can be produced in patients with atrial fibrillation due to diminished conduction from the atria to the ventricles; in part this is mediated through the vagus but in larger doses it results from direct action. A more indirect effect is the occurrence of diuresis which is due to the improvement in the circulation. There is no useful action on the healthy myocardium and digitalis is of no benefit, therefore, where the impediment to the circulation is a mechanical one (e.g. valve stenosis or regurgitation) unless this is complicated by secondary myocardial failure. Unfortunately, the margin between the dose required to achieve the desired therapeutic response and that which leads to toxic effects is small.

Therapeutic use. Digitalis glycosides have their greatest use in the patient with myocardial failure and atrial fibrillation. It is of value also in the management of either of these disorders alone. When used in patients with atrial fibrillation the response of the ventricular rate is usually a convenient index as to the adequacy of treatment. In patients with sinus rhythm it is necessary to give the drug until the desired therapeutic result is obtained or until evidence of toxicity necessitates reduction of dosage.

Digitalis is also of value in the management of other arrhythmias particularly as a prophylaxis against paroxysms of supraventricular tachycardia in young subjects. In atrial flutter it may convert the rhythm to atrial fibrillation and then control the ventricular rate; sometimes it may succeed in increasing the degree of atrioventricular block without change of rhythm, thereby controlling the tachycardia, but more often this is not achieved before serious toxic effects are apparent. Rather surprisingly digitalis may also abolish ventricular or supraventricular ectopic beats, even though in toxic doses it may stimulate them. Digitalis is often ineffective in slowing the heart rate when infection, hyperthyroidism or anxiety are responsible for the tachycardia.

In general, older patients require less digitalis than younger ones; impairment of renal function reduces excretion and therefore the required dose; potassium depletion, most commonly the result of diuretic therapy, potentiates the toxicity of digitalis and this must be watched for in patients on diuretics.

Digoxin has the same actions as digitoxin or prepared digitalis but it is absorbed more rapidly and has a quicker onset of action. It is also available for intramuscular or intravenous injection; the latter is to be preferred as the preparation is irritating and absorption from an intramuscular site is less reliable. By mouth it takes effect in about an hour and peak activity is reached in 6 to 7 hours; by injection onset of effect may be detected in 10 to 15 minutes and the full effect is obtained by 2 hours. After stopping the drug the effect lasts for several days.

Because of its more rapid onset of action digoxin has especial value in the urgent treatment of left heart failure with uncontrolled atrial fibrillation. It is also particularly useful in the management of infants in heart failure where its greater flexibility of use is an advantage.

For rapid effect the usual adult oral loading dose is 1·0 to 1·5 mg followed by 0·25 to 0·5 mg every 6 hours until the desired therapeutic response is achieved. Maintenance usually requires 0·25 mg once to thrice daily. Intravenously 0·5 to 1·0 mg may be given, provided no digitalis preparation has been given in the previous two weeks; if digitalis has been given, not more than 0·25 mg should be given at any one time and at least two hours should elapse between each injection for its effect to be assessed.

For children the loading dose can be calculated on the basis of 0·025 mg per kg bodyweight, either by mouth or injection every 6 hours, adjusted to an appropriate maintenance dose when the desired response is achieved. The administration of small fractional doses is facilitated by the availability of tablets of 0·0625 mg, i.e. one-quarter of the normal 0·25 mg tablet.

Contraindications and side effects. Although theoretically digitalis should not be given to patients with ectopic beats, ventricular arrhythmias or early after myocardial infarction, because of its known potentiating effect on depolarisation, in practice it should not be withheld on these grounds if its use is otherwise indicated.

Gastrointestinal disturbances, anorexia, nausea, vomiting, and sometimes diarrhoea, are usually the first manifestations of digitalis toxicity. Other, less common, non-cardiac manifestations include headache, facial pain, drowsiness, mental confusion, and blurring of vision and, rarely, disturbances of colour vision, so that objects seen by the patient take on a yellow or green hue.

The more serious toxic effects of the digitalis are related to its action on the heart. Ectopic beats, usually ventricular and characteristically coupled to the preceding normal beat are common. In some cases they occur so regularly that they produce pulsus bigeminus which can be readily recognised clinically. When this is not so it is important in patients with atrial fibrillation to ensure that the increased rate and irregularity of the heart beat is not misinterpreted as indicating a lack of control of the atrial fibrillation necessitating an increased dose. Patients previously in sinus rhythm may develop paroxysmal atrial tachycardia with varying atrioventricular block; the continued or increased administration of digitalis in these situations is likely to be fatal. Ventricular tachycardia and later ventricular fibrillation are the usual fatal disturbances of rhythm. Other effects are sinus bradycardia and increased atrioventricular block, at first only detectable on the electrocardiogram but later leading to slowing of the ventricular rate.

Prepared digitalis (Digitalis leaf)

Pharmacological action. As for digoxin.

Prepared digitalis is the dried leaf of the Foxglove, Digitalis purpurea, adjusted by dilution to a standard activity ascertained by biological assay. It contains a number of glycosides.

Therapeutic uses. The usual initial leading dose for an adult is between 1·0 and 1·5 g. given in divided doses over 24 hours; maintenance usually requires 100 to 200 mg daily. It is readily absorbed but its full effect takes some hours to develop; it is slowly excreted and once established the effect may take several days or even weeks to wear off. Now that pure glycoside preparations, which do not require biological assay, are readily available, prepared digitalis is little used.

Contraindications and side effects. As for digoxin.

Digitoxin

Pharmacological action. As for digoxin.

Digitoxin is a crystalline glycoside obtained from the leaves of several species of Digitalis.

Therapeutic use. Digitoxin has properties which are almost identical with those of prepared digitalis, including its slow onset of action and the persistence of its effect. Digitoxin is the most potent (weight for weight) of the cardiac glycosides and the most persistent in its effect; accumulation with prolonged administration may therefore be a problem. There is some clinical evidence that the gastrointestinal side effects are less pronounced than with some other glycosides. In general, however, its slow onset of effect and persistence outweigh this slight advantage and, although widely used in some countries, it would seem to be less convenient than digoxin.

Owing to its high potency the initial loading dose is about 1·0 mg in divided dose and the maintenance dose is between 0·05 and 0·2 mg daily. Preparations for intravenous administration are available but the onset of the effect when given by this route is no faster than when it is given by mouth.

Contraindications and side effects. As for digoxin.

Lanatoside C

Pharmacological action. As for digoxin.

Deslanoside is desacetyl-lanatoside C and is the active material used for intravenous preparations corresponding to the orally administered lanatoside C. Their properties are virtually identical. Lanatoside C is a glycoside obtained from the leaf of Digitalis lanata.

Therapeutic use. These preparations have virtually the same uses as digoxin but have a more rapid onset of action (10 minutes) and a more rapid clearance. They are also reputed to have a larger margin between the therapeutic and toxic dose. For these reasons the intravenous preparation particularly is sometimes of use in rapidly changing situations.

The initial loading dose of lanatoside C given by mouth is about 1·0 to 1·5 mg with a daily maintenance dose of 0·25–0·75 mg daily for adults and a loading dose of 0·25 to 0·05 mg per lb bodyweight for children. For deslanoside given intravenously, the corresponding doses are, for adults 0·8 to 1·2 mg followed by 0·4 mg doses every 2–4 hours as required and, for children 0·01 mg per lb bodyweight.

Contraindications and side effects. As for digoxin.

Aminophylline

Pharmacological action. Aminophylline is a mixture of theophylline and ethylenediamine; the latter helps to improve the solubility of the theophylline and also increases its pharmacological activity. The principal effect of aminophylline is to relax the tone of involuntary muscle, especially of the bronchial tree. It lowers the venous pressure in patients with congestive heart failure. It has a weak diuretic action and also appears to increase the sensitivity of the respiratory centre to increasing carbon dioxide tension.

Therapeutic use. When administered by intravenous injection it has a very rapid beneficial effect on bronchospasm. It is probably most often used for severe bronchial asthma but because of its combination of effects it is of great value in the management of cardiac asthma. The usual dose is 250 mg in 10 ml of solution injected *slowly*.

Aminophylline is not satisfactorily given by mouth because it is a gastric irritant. Several proprietary preparations of aminophylline or closely related substances have been developed to permit oral use; in general they do not have the same potency as the injected drug. It is well absorbed through the rectal mucosa so that, in the form of suppositories, patients can use it for the prevention or relief of attacks of paroxysmal nocturnal dyspnoea. In the UK the suppositories normally contain 360 mg but in the USA they are available with 125, 250 or 500 mg.

Contraindications and side effects. Side effects have been most commonly associated with too-rapid injection; this may lead to restlessness, palpitation, dizziness, nausea, or hypotension. Sudden death has been reported following intravenous injection in normal doses and again this has been associated with rapid injection.

Serious toxic effects appear to have been reported most frequently in children, which suggests that in them its use requires greater caution than in adults.

Quinidine

Pharmacological action. Quinidine is the dextro-rotatory stereo-isomer of quinine. Its principal therapeutic effect is prolongation of the refractory period of cardiac muscle, thereby reducing the rate at which successive contractions can occur. It does, however, have a powerful general depressive action on the myocardium, reducing excitability, contractility and conduction, and it also has some atropine-like action, reducing vagal tone.

Therapeutic use. Quinidine is a potent cardiac-depressant anti-arrhythmic drug, although considered by many to be too toxic for common use. The recent introduction of other less dangerous substances and the advent of the electric-shock correction of arrhythmias have now reduced its usefulness. It may, however, still be the most effective drug in some patients, especially if the arrhythmia is supraventricular. It is often effective in correcting or preventing atrial or ventricular tachyarrhythmias and in abolishing atrial or ventricular ectopic beats. When used for the treatment of supraventricular tachycardias (e.g. atrial flutter) with some degree of atrioventricular block, digitalis should be given first to avoid a sudden, possibly dangerous, increase in ventricular rate which can result from one-to-one conduction developing as the rate of the supraventricular focus is slowed.

Although quinidine may be given intravenously with the protection of electrocardiographic control in urgent cases, e.g. to stop ventricular tachycardia when the patient's life is threatened, it is usually given by mouth. The desired therapeutic response is commonly obtained with a blood level of about 6–8 mg/l. Blood levels above 10 mg/l are associated with a high incidence of toxic effects. The effects of the drug are not, however, uniformly related to the blood level and electrocardiographic monitoring of the response is an alternative way of controlling the dose; the drug may be given until some prolongation of the PR interval and QT time are apparent and changes in the ST segment and T waves occur. An increase in these effects and a widening of the QRS complex are evidence of excessive dosage. Various dose schedules have been described using repeated doses at short intervals to build up higher blood levels each day on top of the residue left from the previous day; a common one uses 0·3 g. or 0·4 g. every 2 hours for 5 doses on successive days for about 3 or 4 days; if necessary the individual dose may be increased to 0·5 g. on the fourth or fifth day and to 0·6 g. on the sixth day. Before starting full therapeutic doses a test dose of 0·2 g. should be given to detect any hypersensitivity.

Contraindications and side effects. Quinidine is absolutely contraindicated by a history of serious reaction to the drug and is given with an increased risk to patients with heart block, or bundle branch block, severe congestive cardiac failure and renal failure, especially in the presence of hyperkalaemia. Individuals may show hypersensitivity to the drug by developing tinnitus, vertigo, blurring of vision or blindness, headache, confusion, rashes, bronchospasm, gastrointestinal disturbances, fever, collapse with hypotension or death from ventricular fibrillation. These reactions may also occur as dose-related side-effects; thrombocytopenic purpura has also been reported. Increase of the width of the QRS complex by more than 25 per cent of its control value, the development of bundle branch block, of second degree or complete heart block, of ventricular ectopic beats, or atrial standstill are all indications of cardiac toxicity and call for withdrawal of the drug before ventricular tachycardia, fibrillation or asystole occur.

Procainamide

Pharmacological action. Procainamide hydrochloride, has a depressant action on the myocardium, diminishing the excitability, conductivity and contractility of both atrium and ventricle, and prolonging the refractory period of the atrium.

Therapeutic use. It is chiefly of use in suppressing ventricular ectopic beats or arrhythmias; it has some effect on atrial arrhythmias and may even convert atrial fibrillation to sinus rhythm, but it is less successful in the management of supraventricular arrhythmias. For the rapid correction of serious arrhythmias, such as ventricular tachycardia, it may be given intravenously but caution is required as it can precipitate depression of myocardial activity with severe hypotension and sometimes the initiation of ventricular fibrillation. It is more safely given by mouth and ,when used for the correction of a rhythm disturbance, the dose is 1·0 g. followed by 0·25 to 1·0 g. every four to six hours. For the long-term prevention of ectopic beats the usual dose is 500 mg every four to six hours. Larger doses are sometimes required. When used intravenously the dose for the control of ventricular arrhythmias is 0·2 to 1·0 g. injected slowly in dilute solution.

Contraindications and side effects. Procainamide antagonises the action of sulphonamides. It should be avoided in patients subject to bronchial asthma and those known to be hypersensitive to it, in patients with renal failure and those with conduction defects of the heart.

Reported side effects include anorexia, nausea, vomiting and diarrhoea, with large oral doses, and severe hypotension when given intravenously. Prolonged or repeated administration may lead to a syndrome resembling systemic lupus erythematosus, leucopenia, granulocytopenia or, rarely, fatal agranulocytosis. Abdominal pain, hepatomegaly with evidence of liver damage, confusion, pruritis and hyper-sensitivity with fever and urticaria have also been described.

Lignocaine (Lidocaine, USA)

Pharmacological action. Although primarily used for its local anaesthetic action, lignocaine decreases cardiac excitability. It differs, however, in having little or no depressant effect on myocardial contractility.

Therapeutic use. Lignocaine is not effective when given by mouth and is more useful in the treatment of ventricular rhythm disorders. Given intravenously it is used to suppress ventricular ectopic beats or to arrest and prevent ventricular tachycardia, especially after myocardial infarction or cardiac surgery. It may be given as a single dose of 1–2 mg per kg of bodyweight or by continuous intravenous infusion at a rate of 1–2 mg per minute.

Contraindications and side effects. Lignocaine should be used with caution in the presence of heart block as it can give rise to asystole. The development of serious tachycardia due to the development of 1:1 conduction as may happen with quinidine (see above) when used in the presence of atrial flutter has been reported. The earliest side effects are drowsiness, euphoria and muscular fasciculation; larger doses may produce hypotension, apprehension, confusion, nausea, vomiting, convulsions and ultimately respiratory and circulatory collapse.

Phenytoin sodium (Sodium diphenylhydantoin, USA)

Pharmacological action. In addition to its anticonvulsant action, phenytoin has been shown to have some anti-arrhythmic effect on the heart. It differs from quinidine and other similarly acting drugs, in showing a stimulant effect on the vagus, slowing atrioventricular conduction and the sinus rate.

Therapeutic use. It is said to be most effective in correcting supraventricular and ventricular arrhythmias resulting from digitalis intoxication and to be of use in preventing paroxysmal arrhythmias. It is not effective in the correction of atrial flutter or fibrillation. The true value of this drug as an anti-arrhythmic agent still remains to be determined.

It may be administered intravenously as a single dose of 250 mg (or 5 mg per kg bodyweight), injected slowly, followed by maintenance doses of 200–400 mg orally, or by intramuscular injecion.

Contraindications and side effects. As it may itself produce bradycardia or atrioventricular block it should not be used when either of these are already present.

Intravenous injection can produce hypotension. Prolonged administration can, of course, produce the toxic effects which are better known in relation to its use as an anticonvulsant.

Propranolol

Pharmacological action. Propranolol is one of a series of compounds with structures related to that of the natural catecholamines, synthesised in a search for a substance which would block the effect of the stimulation of the β-sympathetic receptors. It slows the sinus rate and reduces myocardial contractility to some extent in the resting state but has a more obvious effect in reducing the tachycardia and increase in cardiac output which normally occurs in response to exercise. The subsequent demonstration that propranolol was a racemic mixture of stereoisomers, each of which has slightly different effects, and the preparation of other clinically related substances, each with its own differing spectrum of effects, suggests that the hypothetical concept of β-receptor blockade is an over-simplification; nonetheless, the observed effects mentioned above remain true. In addition, propranolol seems to have some non-specific anti-arrhythmic action resembling that of quinidine.

Therapeutic use. Propranolol found its first application as an antiarrhythmic agent; it is effective in abolishing ectopic beats occurring during anaesthesia and, with digitalis, will often reduce the ventricular rate in atrial fibrillation when digitalis alone fails to do so. It is very effective in controlling sinus tachycardia related to anxiety. It has also been found useful in controlling arrhythmias induced by digitalis intoxication and in hyperthyroidism, where the cardiovascular disturbance is mediated by sympathetic over-activity. It is an effective antidote to tachycardia or rhythm disturbance induced by sympathetic amines therapeutically administered or produced spontaneously by a phaeochromocytoma.

Its effect of impairing myocardial contractility led to its trial in the management of patients with hypertrophic obstructive cardiomyopathy (muscular subaortic stenosis) and of patients with Fallot's tetralogy subject to cyanotic attacks, whose right ventricular outflow obstruction was presumably variable due to a muscular mechanism at infundibular level; in both groups it has provided of value in some cases.

For the above purposes it is usually given orally three or four times a day in doses from 10 to 40 mg each; initially the full desired effect is often obtained by a small dose but it is commonly necessary subsequently to increase this to maintain the response. In acute situations, and when used under anaesthesia, it may be given by intravenous injection; the initial dose then should be only 1–2 mg given slowly, followed by further doses, if required, as the effect of the drug can be assessed; it is recommended, particularly in patients with recent myocardial infarction, that intravenous administration should be preceded by 1–2 mg atropine injected intravenously or bradycardia may occur.

The reduction by propranolol of the normal increase in the cardiac output on exercise suggested that it might be of value in the treatment of angina pectoris by limiting the myocardial demand for oxygen. It has been found to be of considerable value in this respect but maintenance of the response is usually dependent upon considerable increases in the dose up to levels of over 80 mg four times a day. More recently, propranolol has been reported to be of value in the treatment of hypertension.

Contraindications and side effects. Because of its action on the sympathetic nervous control of the bronchiolar musculature it should not be given, or used only with great caution, in patients subject to asthma or bronchospasm of any cause. Because of its myocardial depressant effect, whether this is produced by a direct quinidine-like action or by blockade of a sympathetic drive, it should not be used in patients with myocardial failure or heart block. Even in patients with no clinical evidence of myocardial failure beforehand, propranolol administration has been held responsible for its development subsequently, especially when given on a long-term basis in high doses, usually for the control of angina pectoris. Intravenous administration, especially if the initial dose is rather large (10 mg or more), has been followed by hypotension, extreme bradycardia and occasionally the precipitation of ventricular fibrillation.

Propranolol may also cause nausea, vomiting, diarrhoea, lassitude, depression or insomnia; these effects are reduced by initial low dosage. Less commonly it has produced rashes, non-thrombocytopenic purpura, hallucinations and paraesthesiae.

Glyceryl trinitrate

Pharmacological action. Several organic nitrites and nitrates have a direct action on involuntary muscle, producing relaxation; this effect results in widespread vasodilatation. The distribution and degree of this varies with different compounds but in the case of glyceryl trinitrate is widespread and includes the coronary arterial vessels, but with relatively little effect on the skin vessels. Recent studies have demonstrated that it produces a reduction in the resistance of the coronary circulation but that this is offset by the fall in blood pressure which results from the more generalised vasodilatation so that the myocardial blood flow is diminished; the fall in systemic blood pressure, however, is such that the myocardial work is decreased by a proportion which is greater than that of the reduction of myocardial blood flow. The net result is an increase in myocardial blood flow relative to its work.

Therapeutic use. Glyceryl trinitrate, in the form of 0·5 mg tablets allowed to dissolve in the mouth so that it is absorbed through the oral mucosa, is used for the prevention and relief of angina pectoris. It acts within two or three minutes and the effect lasts for 15 to 30 minutes. Repeated use leads to the development of tolerance but a cessation of use for a few days re-establishes the normal effect.

Contraindications and side effects. Glyceryl trinitrate causes a rise in intraocular tension, so should be avoided in patients with glaucoma. It also causes widespread dilatation of the blood vessels of the head and neck and in some individuals this results in distressing headache or throbbing in the head; it should be used with caution in patients with cerebrovascular disease, intracranial lesions or recent head injury. In some patients the hypotensive effect produces a sensation of syncope which may be accompanied by nausea or vomiting.

Amyl nitrite

Pharmacological action. Similar to glyceryl trinitrate but with a greater effect on the skin vessels, especially of the face and neck.

Therapeutic use. Amyl nitrite is a highly volatile liquid administered by inhalation of the vapour released by crushing a glass capsule containing 0·2 ml of the liquid. It has an effect in about 10 seconds which lasts only 2–3 minutes. Its penetrating odour and the abruptness and intensity of the vasodilatation of the head and face make it objectionable to many patients.

Contraindications and side effects. As for glyceryl trinitrate.

Sorbide nitrate (Isosorbide dinitrate, *USA***)**

Pharmacological action. As for glyceryl trinitrate.

Therapeutic use. When given as a 10 mg tablet dissolved in the mouth its effect is produced in about 10 to 15 minutes and lasts up to 4 hours. With this slower, but more prolonged action it is of little use for the immediate relief of angina pectoris but is recommended as a prophylactic; it is widely used for this purpose in the USA but the reported trials have mostly been uncontrolled and the results have been conflicting.

Pentaerythritol

Pharmacological action. As for glyceryl trinitrate.

Therapeutic use. When given by mouth pentaerythritol tetranitrate produces some fall in the blood pressure after about an hour, which lasts for about 5 hours. It is therefore of no value in the treatment of the acute attack of angina pectoris. It is commonly used as a prophylactic agent although many trials have failed to show any statistically significant benefit. The dose is from 20 to 30 mg.

Dipyridamole

Pharmacological action. Extensive studies in experimental animals and in man have established that dipyridamole has a remarkably selective, but powerful, vasodilator action on the coronary blood vessels, leading to a significant increase in coronary blood flow. It also appears to have an effect in inhibiting platelet clumping.

Therapeutic use. The pharmacological action of dipyridamole led to the expectation that it would be of value in the treatment of ischaemic heart disease; so far no study has shown that it is of any benefit in that condition. It can be given by mouth in a dose of 25 to 50 mg two or three times daily or by slow intravenous injection in a dose of 10 to 20 mg.

Contraindications and side effects. There do not appear to be any contraindications to its use; it may cause anorexia or nausea, headache, dizziness, or faintness and occasionally, after intravenous injection, facial flushing or some fall in the blood pressure.

Prenylamine

Pharmacological action. Like dipyridamole, prenylamine lactate has been shown to have a powerful coronary vascular dilating effect. It also has a slight hypotensive action which is probably mediated by an antagonistic effect against sympathetic activity.

Therapeutic use. The combination of coronary vasodilatation and sympathetic blockade suggests that this drug should be of value in the treatment of angina pectoris. Several trials have reported its successful use as a prophylactic agent in a dose of 60 mg two to four times a day.

Contraindications and side effects. Prenylamine is contraindicated in the presence of conduction defects, heart failure, or hepatic disease. Patients already receiving hypotensive agents may require some reduction in the dose whilst receiving prenylamine. Gastric intolerance has been reported occasionally when the drug is first administered; rashes rarely occur.

Cholestyramine

Pharmacological action. Cholestyramine is a basic anion–exchange resin which binds bile acids in the intestine and thereby prevents their resorption and interferes with the absorption of other lipids.

Therapeutic use. In total daily doses of between 12 and 15 g. cholestyramine has been shown to reduce the blood–cholesterol levels in patients with hypercholesterolaemia and has been used to correct this biochemical deviation in the hope of reducing the risk of development of atheroma. It is also said to be effective in relieving itching in obstructive jaundice.

Contraindications and side effects. It may produce gastrointestinal discomfort.

Clofibrate

Pharmacological action. Clofibrate lowers elevated serum triglyceride and cholesterol levels by its effects upon low-density β-lipoproteins. These effects appear to result from the binding of clofibrate to specific sites on the plasma proteins which in turn leads to a redistribution between the plasma and liver of several factors which affect the blood-lipid pattern. It also seems to correct a number of factors which produce the hypercoagulability often associated with atherosclerotic disease.

Therapeutic uses. Prolonged administration is used in patients with atherosclerosis, especially if this is manifest by clinical evidence of coronary heart disease, cerebral or peripheral vascular disease and those with hyperlipidaemia or diabetic arteriopathy in the hope of reducing progression of vascular disease. The drug is introduced gradually and is then maintained at 20 to 30 mg per kg bodyweight daily in divided doses.

Contraindications and side effects. Clofibrate should not be given during pregnancy, or to patients with impaired renal or hepatic function. It potentiates the action of anticoagulant drugs and, in some patients, of insulin so that it should be introduced cautiously to patients receiving these. It may cause nausea, gastrointestinal discomfort, drowsiness or produce rashes; a gain in weight frequently follows its administration. A rise in serum transaminases and a fall in alkaline phosphatase levels may occur but are probably related to the action of the drug rather than to hepatotoxicity.

Isoprenaline (Isoproterenol, *USA*)

Pharmacological action. Isoprenaline is a potent stimulator of the β-receptors of the sympathetic nervous system. It increases the heart rate improves atrio-ventricular conduction, increases myocardial contractility and produces predominant vasodilation in the systemic circulation.

Therapeutic use. It is of considerable value in improving myocardial function in patients who have had recent myocardial infarction or undergone major cardiac surgery and thereby leads to improved tissue perfusion. For this purpose it is infused intravenously as 2 to 5 mg diluted in 500 ml of 5 per cent dextrose at a rate of from 2 to 50 drops per minute, carefully controlled and adjusted according to the response of the patient whose electrocardiogram should be under continuous oscilloscope observation. In the form of tablets of 30 mg contained in a slow release base it can be given by mouth to increase the idioventricular rate or improve the conduction in patients with complete heart block.

Contraindications and side effects. Isoprenaline should not be given to patients with hyperthyroidism or who have any form of ventricular arrhythmia. It can provoke tachycardia, ectopic beats and ventricular fibrillation. Headache, palpitations, anginal pain, flushing, apprehension, tremor, nausea and weakness are common side effects of overdosage.

Atropine

Pharmacological action. In relation to the cardiovascular system atropine blocks the inhibiting effect of vagal activity on the sinus and atrioventricular nodes. If the heart is affected by increased vagal tone atropine increases the heart rate and reduces the atrioventricular conduction time.

Therapeutic use. It is the specific treatment for vagally mediated bradycardia with or without atrioventricular conduction defect such as may occur from digitalis intoxication or reflexly after myocardial infarction, DC shock correction of arrhythmias, or in response to procedures such as aortic catheterization or cardiac puncture. For this purpose it can be given by intravenous injection of between 0·25 and 1·5 mg.

Contraindications and side effects. See above.

Calcium chloride

Pharmacological action. In relation to the cardiovascular system it is a powerful stimulator of myocardial contractility.

Therapeutic use. The effect of calcium chloride is transient so that it is of no value for long-term treatment but a slow injection of 0·5 to 2 g. intravenously will often restore the contractility of an asystolic ventricle or improve that of a fibrillating ventricle so as to permit successful electrical defibrillation.

Contraindications and side effects. Calcium chloride should not be used if digitalis intoxication is a possible cause of the arrhythmia. Calcium chloride is irritating to the tissues so that care must be exercised during intravenous injection.

This chapter was written by Dr D. C. Deuchar (Physician to the Cardiac Dept, Guy's Hospital) and edited by Prof. J. R. Trounce.

Category 7

Drugs Used in the Treatment of Hypertensive Disease

RAUWOLFIA ALKALOIDS

This group of alkaloids are mild hypotensive agents. They may be used either as various crude fractions or as the pure alkaloids (reserpine, rescinnamine, deserpidine). Reserpine is the most widely used.

Reserpine

Pharmacological action. Reserpine lowers blood pressure by reducing the activity of the sympathetic nervous system and also by a tranquillizing and depressing action on the brain. Reserpine depletes catecholamines in both the peripheral sympathetic nervous system and in the brain and it seems probable its effects are due to this depletion.

Therapeutic uses. Reserpine in doses of up to 0·25 mg twice daily has a moderate blood pressure lowering action which is unrelated to posture, and which is due to fall in peripheral resistance. It is well absorbed from the intestine but it is usually four or five days before it begins to lower the blood pressure and it may be a week or two before it becomes fully effective. Likewise its activity will continue for several days after stopping the drug. At this dosage level side effects can be troublesome and a lower dose (0·25 mg daily) may be used, combined with a diuretic.

There are a number of other preparations available which contain reserpine or related alkaloids. They include:

Methoserpedine, 10 mg
Rescinnamine, 0·35 mg } equivalent to 0·25 mg of Reserpine
Deserpedine, 0·5 mg

There is no evidence that they have any advantage over reserpine.
The other actions of reserpine can be grouped:
(a) Sympatholytic effects: including bradycardia, nasal stuffiness and extrasystoles. There may also be increased gastrointestinal motor

activity with a raised gastric acid secretion and occasionally peptic ulceration and diarrhoea.

(b) Central effects can be troublesome. Some drowsiness and general lack of 'go' with decreased libido is common, and occasionally a psychotic depression develops. With large doses a Parkinson-like state can be produced.

In addition, patients may show weight gain due to fluid retention.

Contraindications and side effects. Reserpine should not be used in depressed patients and should be used with care in those with intestinal disease, particularly peptic and ulcerative colitis. In a patient on reserpine, a general anaesthetic may provoke a considerable fall in blood pressure, though this is not universally accepted.

Hydrallazine

Pharmacological action. Hydrallazine [1] produces a widespread vasodilatation with a fall in blood pressure which is not usually affected by posture. The greatest fall is in the diastolic pressure. This is accompanied by a rise in pulse rate and cardiac output which to some extent neutralises the hypotensive action of the drug. How this rise in cardiac output is achieved is not known but it is possible that hydrallazine reflexly augments the actions of the adrenergic nervous system.

Hydrallazine is well absorbed and the drug is largely metabolised.

Therapeutic uses. Hydrallazine is a mild blood pressure lowering agent and its use is limited by the high incidence of side effects. The initial dose is 10 mg four times daily, and this is gradually increased to a total of 100–200 mg daily. In order to prevent the rise in pulse rate and cardiac output which accompanies its use hydrallazine may be combined with propranolol (see above). It increases renal blood flow and is therefore said to be particularly useful in hypertension complicating renal disease.

Contraindications and side effects. Headaches are particularly common at the start of treatment, but usually disappear after a week or so of continued treatment. They may be accompanied by nausea and diarrhoea. In the higher dose range (over 400 mg daily) and after prolonged treatment about 10 per cent of patients show a rheumatoid-like syndrome, sometimes accompanied by a positive L.E. phenomena. This may take a considerable time to subside after stopping the drug.

Hydrallazine may also produce skin rashes and rarely a peripheral neuropathy.

The rise in pulse rate and output caused by hydrallazine may precipitate anginal pain in those with coronary disease. Under these circumstances it should be combined with propranolol.

THE GANGLION BLOCKERS

Pharmacological action. The ganglion blockers were the first effective blood pressure lowering agents. They interfere with transmission at the relay ganglia of both the adrenergic and cholinergic nervous system. At these sites they compete with acetylcholine and thus prevent depolarisation of the membrane of the postsynaptic nerve cells.

The actions of these drugs can be grouped according to the system involved:

1. *Cardiovascular system.* Loss of adrenergic tone leads to arterial and venous vasodilatation. This causes pooling of blood with a decreased venous return to the heart and a fall in cardiac output. The drop in cardiac output and the arteriolar dilatation are responsible for the fall in blood pressure which is largely postural (i.e. only seen on standing and abolished by lying flat).

2. *Gastrointestinal.* Loss of cholinergic activity causes a dry mouth, slows intestine transit, and leads to constipation and occasionally ileus.

3. *Genitourinary.* Retention may occur especially if there is some bladder neck obstruction and impotence is an occasional complication.

4. *Eyes.* Pupils may dilate with paralysis of accommodation.

These drugs are largely excreted by the kidney and with impaired renal function, accumulation will occur.

Therapeutic uses. Although they are potent hypotensive agents, the widespread pharmacological effect of these drugs, and the fact that the fall in blood pressure is postural, has led to their being replaced by other agents and they are now rarely used.

The chief individual ganglion blockers available are:

Hexamethonium bromide was the prototype drug. It is irregularly and poorly absorbed from the intestine and was not therefore very satisfactory for the long-term treatment of hypertension.

Pentolinium tartrate is slightly better absorbed orally, but is now largely used in hypertensive crises when it is given by subcutaneous injection. The initial dose is 2·5 mg (1·25 mg in the elderly) and then a further 1·0 mg is given every fifteen minutes until a satisfactory fall in blood pressure is produced. (Note the blood pressure must be taken sitting or standing.)

Mecamylamine is well absorbed from the intestine and the initial oral dose is 2·5 mg twice daily. This is increased every four days until a satisfactory fall in blood pressure is produced. Mecamylamine is only slowly excreted in an alkaline urine and because of this should not be combined with acetazolamide. In addition to the side effects of ganglion blockade, mecamylamine may produce tremor and weakness due to an action on voluntary muscle.

Pempidine is also absorbed and the initial dose is 2·5 mg three times a day and increased as required.

Trimetaphan is a very rapidly acting ganglion blocker. It is given by intravenous infusion in a 1 in 1000 solution. Its effects pass off rapidly after stopping infusion. It is largely used to produce controlled postural hypotension.

Contraindications. Ganglion blockers should be used with care or not at all in patients where a sudden fall in blood pressure could be dangerous. This will include those with severe myocardial or cerebral ischaemia.

In patients with renal failure a blood urea of over 100 mg%, usually contraindicates as a large fall in blood pressure may cause a further disastrous deterioration in renal function and there is also the problem of impaired excretion.

Patients on these drugs are unduly sensitive to sympathomemetic amines.

THE ADRENERGIC BLOCKING AGENTS

(a) THOSE BLOCKING THE POST GANGLIONIC NERVES [2]

This group of drugs is the most widely used to lower blood pressure. They all produce this effect by interfering in some way with the release of noradrenaline at the adrenergic nerve ending. In general, they also cause a fall in blood pressure, which is largely postural. This is largely due to loss of vasomotor tone causing peripheral pooling of blood with decreased venous return and a lowered cardiac output. Prolonged treatment may result in some increase in blood volume and thus some decrease in efficiency of the hypotensive agent [3].

They all have side effects which are referable to adrenergic blockade. There are however minor differences in both the duration of action and in the incidence of side effects.

The main drugs of this type in use at present are:

Guanethidine

Pharmacological action. Guanethidine decreases a release of noradrenaline at adrenergic nerve endings. If injected intravenously it causes a transient rise in blood pressure, because it inhibits re-uptake of noradrenaline by nerve endings. Guanethidine also causes some depletion of peripheral noradrenaline stores. It is only moderately well absorbed from the intestines and is only slowly excreted by the kidneys, and it is several days before a single dose is cleared from the body. This means that one dose daily is adequate.

Therapeutic uses. Guanethidine is given initially in a dose of 10 mg in the morning. The dose is increased at weekly intervals until a satisfactory control of blood pressure is produced, usually with around 20–60 mg daily. The rather prolonged action of guanethidine makes it difficult to control the blood pressure if it varies widely throughout the day. Tolerance does not usually develop to any marked extent with guanethidine, but can be due to sodium and water retention and is controlled by using a diuretic.

Contraindications and side effects. Diarrhoea is the most troublesome side effect but can be controlled with codeine phosphate or with the addition of a ganglion blocking agent. Bradycardia is usual but is not important. Other results of adrenergic blockade are failure of ejaculation and parotid pain.

As with the ganglion blockers guanethidine must be used with great care in those with marked cerebral or myocardial ischaemia or in renal failure.

Guanoxan

Pharmacological action. Guanoxan is a combination of the guanethidine ring with benzodioxane. It blocks release of noradrenaline and also depletes peripheral stores. In addition, presumably due to its benzodioxane moity it has some direct blocking action on circulating adrenaline and noradrenaline. The fall in blood pressure is postural but less markedly so than guanethidine.

Therapeutic uses. Guanoxan is administered in an initial dose of 20 mg daily and increased every four days as required [4].

Contraindications and side effects. Guanoxan causes diarrhoea and failure of ejaculation. In addition it may cause drowsiness, particularly early in treatment. Changes in liver function tests are not uncommon and occasionally they may be followed by jaundice.

It would seem that the risk of liver damage should limit the use of the drug.

Guanochlor

Pharmacological action. Guanochlor interferes with noradrenaline release and storage and may also interfere with the conversion of dopamine to noradrenaline. It produces a postural fall in blood pressure.

Therapeutic use. Guanochlor is given in an initial dose of 10 mg b.d. [5] and this is increased every third day until a satisfactory fall in blood pressure is produced.

Contraindications and side effects. In a few patients guanochlor causes some urea retention but there does not appear to be any interference with overall renal function. It may also cause salt and water retention and may have to be combined with a diuretic. Guanochlor causes pain in skeletal muscle in a small number of patients; the reason for this is unknown [6]. Other side effects are similar to those of the adrenergic blocking group as a whole.

Bethanidine

Pharmacological action. Bethanidine lowers blood pressure by blocking noradrenaline release from the adrenergic nerve endings. It has no peripheral depleting action and no blocking action on circulating noradrenaline. It is rapidly and well absorbed producing a peak effect within four to five hours. It is excreted via the kidneys and entirely eliminated within about twelve hours.

Therapeutic use. The relatively short action of bethanidine enables the blood pressure to be controlled more flexibly as the dose can be modified to meet fluctuation during the day [7].

The initial dose is 10 mg twice daily and this is increased by adding 5 or 10 mg to each dose until adequate control is obtained. If the blood pressure is very variable during the day bethanidine can be given three or four times daily. Some tolerance may develop.

In severe hypertension it appears to have some synergistic action with methyldopa [8].

Contraindications and side effects. The fall in blood pressure is markedly postural. However, diarrhoea is unusual.

Other side effects are similar to guanethidine, but it occasionally causes depression. It should not be used when a phaeochromocytoma is suspected and should not be combined with the amphetamine group of drugs.

Debrisoquine

Pharmacological action. Debrisoquine prevents release of noradrenaline at adrenergic nerve endings without depleting peripheral stores and produces a postural fall in blood pressure. It is relatively rapid in action and is very similar to bethanidine.

Therapeutic uses. The initial dose is 10 mg twice daily and this is increased every three or four days until a satisfactory fall in blood pressure results.

Contraindications and side effects. Debrisoquine is fairly free of side effects [9]. When they occur they include diarrhoea, failure of ejaculation, muscle weakness and tiredness. Contraindications are the same for any agent which can cause a considerable fall in blood pressure.

(b) THOSE INTERFERING WITH NORADRENALINE SYNTHESIS

Methyldopa

Pharmacological action. Methyldopa differs from all the other drugs which inhibit the adrenergic nervous system. It is believed to be converted to methylnoradrenaline at the adrenergic nerve endings and this substance which is only a weak vasoconstrictor acts as a 'false mediator'. The important result of this is that with methyldopa the fall in blood pressure is almost as great lying as standing.

Methyldopa is well absorbed but its hypotensive effect is delayed for 4–6 hours. It is excreted via the kidneys and about half the dose is cleared from the body in twelve hours, and excretion is complete in 48 hours.

Therapeutic use. Methyldopa is very widely used in the treatment of hypertension. The initial dose is 250 mg twice daily and this is increased every fourth day until a satisfactory response is obtained. The usual dose being 250 mg four times daily. It is not worth giving more than 2·0 g. daily as further increases in dose will not usually increase the hypotensive effect. Methyldopa has a tendency to provoke sodium and water retention and its action can be augmented by combining it with a diuretic.

Contraindications and side effects. Methyldopa produces drowsiness in 20–30 per cent of patients, although this may diminish with continued treatment. Other side effects include dry mouth, nasal congestion and lactation. Marked water retention is rare but can cause oedema. It responds to a diuretic.

Methyldopa can also provoke hypersensitivity phenomena. About 20 per cent of those on long term treatment at high dosage levels develop a positive direct Coombs test [10] and occasionally a frank haemolytic anaemia. Other hypersensitivity phenomena have been described, including drug fever, skin rashes and rarely, liver damage. In patients with renal failure, retention of the drug can give rise to a parkinson-like state.

Methyldopa should therefore not be used in liver disease, and with care in those with impaired renal function.

(c) BETA-ADRENERGIC BLOCKING AGENTS

Propranolol
Pharmacological action. See above.

Therapeutic use. Propranolol has been used with success in hypertension [11]. The fall in blood pressure is not postural. It is tentatively suggested that as a result of β blockade of the heart, transient rises in cardiac output and blood pressure are prevented. The aortic arch baroreceptors become readjusted and the blood pressure is 'set' at a lower level.

The initial dose is 10 mg four times daily and this is increased at fortnightly intervals by 25 per cent of the dose until blood pressure is controlled. It may take two months before the full effect is seen.

Contraindications and side effects. See above.

(d) ALPHA-ADRENERGIC BLOCKING AGENTS (see above)

Phentolamine   Phenoxybenzamine

(e) MONOAMINE-OXIDASE INHIBITORS

Pargyline
Pharmacological action. The drug is a monoamine–oxidase inhibitor and also lowers blood pressure, probably by blocking the post-ganglionic

part of the adrenergic nervous system. The fall in blood pressure is partially postural.

It is only slowly excreted and one dose daily is adequate.

Therapeutic uses. Pargyline [12] is given in an initial dose of 25 mg orally. It takes about two weeks to produce its full effect and the dose is thereafter increased by 10 mg at two-weekly intervals.

Contraindications and side effects. Pargyline has all the side effects and dangers of other MAO inhibitors (see above). These inherent dangers limit its use as a hypertensive agent. It is also contraindicated in liver or kidney failure, in thyrotoxicosis and in pregnancy.

DIURETICS

Pharmacology. A wide variety of diuretics will lower blood pressure. In the early stages of treatment this appears related to the decrease in circulating blood volume which follows naturesis. However, after some weeks treatment both blood volume and cardiac output return to normal but the hypotensive action continues.

Therapeutic use. The fall in blood pressure produced by diuretics is relatively small but they are particularly useful when combined with other hypotensive agents when they increase and smooth out the hypotensive action of these drugs. They may also prevent the development of resistance to some hypotensive drugs, in particular the adrenergic blocking agents.

In theory, the longer-acting diuretics, such as chlorthalidone should be most suitable in hypertension, but in practice any of the benzothiadizines, or even the relatively short-acting frusemide are satisfactory. The choice of diuretics and side effects are considered later.

Diazoxide

Diazoxide is related to the benzothiadiazine diuretics. It is a powerful blood pressure lowering agent when given intravenously, probably by a direct action on the arterial wall. The dose by this route is 5 mg/kg I.V., given undiluted, and it is not so effective if given diluted in an intravenous drip. The fall in blood pressure lasts 6–24 hours.

Unfortunately the drug is not effective orally and further repeated use leads to rise in blood sugar levels. This latter action has been used in the treatment of hypoglycaemia [13].

PERIPHERAL VASODILATORS

Tolazoline

Pharmacological action. Tolazoline produces peripheral vasodilatation, mainly of skin vessels. This is largely due to a direct action on the vessel wall but it is also a weak α receptor blocker. Tolazoline also increases both heart rate and output, and so may actually increase blood pressure. It also stimulates gastric secretion. It is well absorbed and rapidly excreted via the kidneys.

Therapeutic uses. Tolazoline is used in doses of 25–50 mg three times a day in the treatment of peripheral vascular disease. There is no good evidence that it has any benefit in atherosclerotic disease but may help in Raynaud's phenomena.

Contraindications and side effects. Tolazoline may cause tachycardia and cardiac arrhythmias, flushing and diarrhoea. It may also exacerbate peptic ulceration.

It should not be used in heart failure, angina of effort, or in those with peptic ulceration.

Cyclendelate

Pharmacology and therapeutic use. The drug produces vasodilatation by acting directly on the arterial wall. It has been used for peripheral vascular disease and is also claimed to increase cerebral blood flow. There is little evidence that it is of benefit in vascular disease of the limbs or the brain.

The usual dose is 400 mg three times daily. Side effects include flushing, dizziness and headaches.

Inositol nicotinate

A mild vasodilatator. The initial dose is 200 mg four times daily and it can be increased. It appears free of ill effects.

Isoxsuprine

This drug causes a combination of peripheral vasodilatation with an increase in cardiac output. The dose is 10 mg four times daily. Its efficiency in peripheral vascular disease is doubtful.

References

1. Schirger, A., and Spittell, J. A., *Amer. J. Cardiol.* (1962), **9**, 854.
2. Pritchard, B. N. C., Johnston, A. W., Hill, I. D., and Rosenheim, M. L., *Brit. med. J.* (1968), **1**, 135.

3. Romnov-Jersen, V., *Acta med. Scand.* (1963), **174**, 300.
4. Peart, W. S., and MacMahon, M. I., *Brit. med. J.* (1964), **1**, 398.
5. Peart, W. S., and MacMahon, M. I., *ibid.*, 402.
6. Hodge, J. V., *ibid.* (1966), **2**, 981.
7. Montuschi, E., and Pickens, P. T., *Lancet* (1962), **ii**, 897.
8. Breckenridge, A., and Dollery, C. T., *ibid.* (1966), **i**, 1074.
9. Athanassiadis, D., Cranston, W. I., Juel-Jensen, B. F., and Olives, D. O., *Brit. med. J.* (1966), **2**, 732.
10. Carstairs, K. C., Breckenridge, A., Dollery, C. T., and Wolledge, S. M., *Lancet* (1966), **ii**, 133.
11. Pritchard, B. N. C., and Gillam, P. M. S., *Brit. med. J.* (1969), **1**, 7.
12. Moser, M., Brodoff, B., Miller, A., and Goldman, A. G., *Amer. med. Arch.* (1964), **187**, 192.
13. Graber, A. L., Porte, D., and Williams, R. H., *Diabetes* (1966), **15**, 143.

This chapter was written by Professor J. R. Trounce.

Category 8

Diuretics and Cation Exchange Resins

DIURETICS

Diuretics are indicated in any patient who has adequate renal function and who has oedema arising from a central rather than a local cause [1]. They play a major part in the management of cardiac failure and of oedema attributable to a low plasma protein level whether this arises on a nutritional, hepatic, or renal basis. In addition they have a valuable supplementary role in the treatment of hypertension [1, 2] and are sometimes useful in the treatment of acute-on-chronic respiratory failure and of some cases of poisoning.

The power of modern diuretics has diminished the therapeutic value of dietary sodium restriction. This still has a place, however, and its effect may be increased by the oral administration of a cation exchange resin in the potassium, ammonium or calcium phase.

Benzothiadiazines and related drugs

Pharmacological actions and therapeutic use [1]. There are at least twelve drugs of this type in use [1] (Table 1). They differ in their intestinal absorption and diuretic potency and in their solubility in fat which determines their rate of excretion, and duration of action.

In addition there are a number of closely related drugs (Table 2) which have a different heterocyclic moiety but common side chains, similar actions and identical side effects.

All these drugs increase the urinary excretion of sodium and have secondary effects on the excretion of water, chloride and potassium. They are weak inhibitors of carbonic anhydrase and may impair the ability to excrete an acid urine.

Some doubt exists concerning their sites of action on the kidney. Stop-flow studies indicate an effect on the proximal convoluted tubule but recent micropuncture work suggests that the most important action is on the distal convoluted tubule [3]. They are all given orally and, in addition, there is a preparation of chlorothiazide that is suitable for intravenous injection (dose: 500 mg). The shorter acting drugs are

Table 1 The Benzothiadiazines

Approved name		Duration of action (hours)	Dose (mg)
Chlorothiazide		12	500 −2000
Cyclopenthiazide		12	0·25–2·0
Cyclothiazide		24	1·0 −8·0
Bendrofluazide	Bendroflumethiazide (USA)	18	2·5 −10·0
Benzthiazide		12	25 −200
Flumethiazide		12	250 −2000
Hydrochlorothiazide		14	25 −200
Hydroflumethiazide		14	25 −200
Methyclothiazide		24	2·5 −10·0
Polythiazide		48	1·0 −8·0
Teclothiazide		10	110 −220
Trichlormethiazide		24	1·0 −8·0

Table 2 Diuretics which resemble the Benzothiadiazines

Approved name	Duration of action (hours)	Dose (mg)
Chlorthalidone	72	50–200
Clorexolone	48	25–100
Quinethazone	24	50–200
Clopamide	36	20–80

given daily, usually in the mornings, but the longer acting ones need be given only on alternate days.

In addition to their conventional uses, the benzothiadiazines have been shown to lower the urinary excretion of calcium and may prove to be of value in the prevention of renal calculi.

Contraindications and side effects. The benzothiadiazines and related drugs are all fairly safe but have a number of well recognised side effects.

Early in treatment, potassium excretion rises due to the increased amount of sodium available for exchange in the distal tubule. Later, relatively less sodium and more potassium ions appear in the urine and, eventually, potassium may become the major urinary cation with the development of potassium depletion and an extracellular alkalosis. Ultimately oedema may be completely resistant to treatment and the serum sodium concentration falls. Intracellular potassium depletion contributes to this state [4] and it is advisable to stop the diuretic and replace potassium while restricting the intake of sodium and water. Although the serum potassium level is a poor index of potassium depletion, it is worth measuring it regularly in those on prolonged treatment especially with large doses of diuretic. In such patients supplements of potassium chloride are indicated (see below).

Secretion of uric acid by the distal tubule is inhibited with retention of uric acid and the production of hyperuricaemia [1]. Occasionally this is associated with episodes of acute gout which subside when the drug is withdrawn or when uricosuric drugs (e.g. probenecid) are used. Most patients develop some impairment of carbohydrate tolerance and a few become frankly diabetic; improvement occurs on stopping the drug but a few patients continue to require treatment for diabetes. Finally, occasional patients develop thrombocytopaenic purpura, leucopenia, photosensitivity, macular-papular rashes or jaundice.

Frusemide (Furosemide, USA)

Pharmacological actions and therapeutic use. Frusemide has some chemical similarity to the benzothiadiazines but produces a substantially greater diuretic effect [1, 5]. This is not increased by the addition of a benzothiadiazine suggesting that frusemide acts at the same sites in the tubule plus another site which is thought to be the ascending limb of Henle's loop [3]. Absorption from the gut is rapid and complete, and excretion is by the kidney.

A diuresis begins within two minutes of intravenous administration (dose: 20–60 mg) and lasts only two hours. This makes it ideal for the treatment of acute pulmonary oedema.

After oral administration (dose: 40–120 mg) the diuretic effect lasts about four hours. This transient action makes it relatively unsuitable for maintenance therapy unless weaker drugs have proved ineffective. Its great power makes it useful in the treatment of patients with impaired renal function when very large doses (500 mg) may be given.

Contraindications and side effects. The main problems derive from its potency, and it is easy to produce acute hypovolaemia and chronic electrolyte depletion. It is logical to start treatment with a small dose and to take particular care when the oedema is associated with hypoproteinaemia and hypovolaemia. In these circumstances it may be necessary to maintain the blood volume by the intravenous administration of salt poor albumin or an osmotic diuretic (see below). Apart from this, the drug is fairly safe; potassium depletion and hyperuricaemia occur frequently but carbohydrate intolerance is seen less often than with the benzothiadiazines. Leucopenia, thrombocytopenia and diarrhoea have been reported.

Ethacrynic acid

Pharmacological actions and therapeutic use. Chemically this drug differs substantially from frusemide and the benzothiadiazines. It has a powerful diuretic action which is not increased by frusemide and which lasts about eight hours [1, 6]. It is well absorbed from the gut (dose: 50–400 mg) and may also be given intravenously (dose: 50 mg). Excretion is via the kidneys.

Contraindications and side effects. Electrolyte depletion and hypovolaemia are real hazards and it is essential to start treatment with small doses. Potassium supplements are necessary during maintenance therapy. Hyperuricaemia, thrombocytopenia and skin rashes may also occur and there is a rather high incidence of gastro-intestinal symptoms. Patients have been reported who developed deafness when treated with large doses of ethacrynic acid in the presence of renal failure.

Organic mercurials

Pharmacological actions and therapeutic use. These drugs were the first effective diuretics and remain among the most powerful [1]. Unfortunately they are poorly absorbed from the gut and are usually given by intramuscular injection; in view of this inconvenience they have been largely replaced by oral diuretics. They inhibit sodium reabsorption in the proximal convoluted tubule but also act on the distal part of the nephron [3]. Chlormerodrin and mercurophylline may be given orally but are not as powerful as mersalyl and mercaptomerin which are given by injection. Mersalyl Inj. B.P. (dose: 2 ml I.M.) contains a small amount of theophylline which is itself a weak diuretic (see below) but which is included because it improves absorption from the injection site. The action lasts twenty-four hours and it is usual to repeat the dose every 2–4 days. Diuresis is enhanced by the administration of ammonium chloride (dose: 2–6 g. daily). This may be attributable to the chloride ion but it is possible that the acidifying effect releases active mercuric ion within the tubular cell.

Contraindications and side effects. Occasional patients develop hyper-sensitivity reactions with bronchospasm and urticaria. Stomatitis and anorexia may also occur with prolonged courses. Other side effects are rare but include proteinuria, the nephrotic syndrome and acute renal failure. Mercurials are not given to patients with established renal disease and it is advisable to test the urine regularly during treatment. If a patient becomes resistant to mersalyl there is a risk of mercury poisoning and treatment should be stopped. The drug must not be given by intravenous injection. Significant potassium depletion is rare and it is unnecessary to give supplements routinely although it is wise to measure the plasma potassium level occasionally.

Triamterene

Pharmacological actions and therapeutic use. This drug has a relatively weak action and is not given alone. It inhibits sodium/potassium exchange in the distal convoluted tubule and supplements the effect of diuretics which act higher up the nephron. It is given orally, the usual dose being 100–250 mg daily.

Contraindications and side effects. Potassium retention and hyperkalaemia occur frequently, and reversible impairment of renal function may also be seen. Plasma levels of urea and potassium should be measured regularly and the drug should not be given to patients with renal failure. Other side effects include anorexia, abdominal discomfort and skin rashes.

Spironolactone

Pharmacological actions and therapeutic use. The majority of oedematous patients, particularly those with hypoproteinaemia, have evidence of hyperaldosteronism. Spironolactone is a competitive inhibitor of the action of aldosterone and has a weak diuretic effect with conservation of potassium. It is used in combination with drugs acting higher up the nephron and has a definite place in the treatment of resistant oedema when its effect on potassium excretion is particularly valuable. The original preparation was poorly absorbed from the gut and has been replaced by a microcrystalline form which is absorbed better. The dose is 25 mg q.d.s. and it is common to observe a delay of two or three days before the diuretic effect appears. In the treatment of primary hyper-aldosteronism very large (100 mg q.d.s.) doses must be used.

Contraindications and side effects. These are rare but include gynaeco-mastia, hirsutism, headache, mental confusion and drowsiness. Hyper-kalaemia may develop and spironolactone should not be given to patients with renal failure.

Amiloride (MK 870)

This drug is not yet available for general use.

Pharmacological actions and therapeutic use. Chemically it has a minor resemblance to triamterene, and similarly produces a sodium and water diuresis with conservation of potassium [7]. It is a more powerful diuretic and potentiates the action of ethacrynic acid and the benzo-thiadiazines. The oral dose is 10–40 mg daily and the action is complete within twenty-four hours.

Contraindications and side effects. Limited experience has revealed no toxic effects apart from a small rise in the plasma potassium concentration.

Carbonic anhydrase inhibitors

Pharmacological actions and therapeutic use. As diuretics, these drugs [1], which include acetazolamide, ethoxzolamide, methazolamide, and dichlorphenamide, are now only of historic interest. They prevent bicarbonate reabsorption and the excretion of hydrogen ions, leading to an increased excretion of sodium and potassium ions. However, the effect is transient as the development of a metabolic acidosis leads to a fall in the filtered bicarbonate.

Contraindications and side effects. These include potassium depletion, renal calculi, drowsiness, paraesthesiae, thrombocytopenia and skin rashes.

Xanthines

Pharmacological actions and therapeutic use. The xanthines are weak diuretics and are not used alone. Caffeine and theophylline act when given orally but aminophylline, the most effective, is inactivated by gastric acidity and is given either as suppositories (360 mg) or intra-venously (250–500 mg). Aminophylline increases the cardiac output and may be given at the peak of a diuresis produced by other diuretics when it produces a further increase in urine flow.

Contraindications and side effects. Cardiac arrest has been observed following rapid intravenous injection of aminophylline and this drug must therefore be given slowly over several minutes. Despite this precaution, vomiting and hypotension may occur.

OSMOTIC DIURETICS

Mannitol
Pharmacological actions and therapeutic use. Osmotic diuretics are believed to act by increasing the solute load per nephron, which in turn decreases the tubular transit time and the time available for reabsorption of water and electrolytes. Alternatively it is possible that sodium and water reabsorption in the proximal convoluted tubule is limited by the relative hypertonicity of the tubular contents.

Mannitol may be used in the treatment of resistant oedema associated with hypoproteinaemia and hypovolaemia. It is given at the same time as a conventional diuretic and leads to a further increase in urine flow while the patient is protected from the expected fall in blood volume. It also has a place in the treatment of poisoning with drugs such as phenobarbitone and the salicylates, which are filtered at the glomerulus and partially reabsorbed by the tubules. The usual dose is 25–50 g. followed by continuous intravenous administration of 10–20 g./hour, the rate being adjusted according to the response observed.

There is good evidence that under certain circumstances, the preoperative prophylactic administration of mannitol protects patients from the development of acute renal failure. However, the value of mannitol therapy in the treatment of patients with incipient acute renal failure is not yet proved. Providing there are no signs of circulatory overload a formal trial of mannitol is justified; occasionally there is a dramatic response but if there is none, the treatment must be stopped.

Contraindications and side effects. Two principal dangers arise from treatment of this type. Circulatory overload may be avoided by regular observation, careful fluid balance, and the cessation of treatment in the absence of a diuresis. The second danger is of fluid and electrolyte depletion; the composition of the urine passed must be measured and any losses which are not required must be replaced intravenously.

POTASSIUM SUPPLEMENTS

The majority of diuretics produce significant potassium loss and, unless spironolactone, triamterene or amiloride are being used, the administration of potassium supplements should be considered. A high potassium intake in the form of fresh fruit is advisable. However, many potassium rich foods such as milk and meat extracts are also rich in sodium and may be contraindicated. Potassium depletion is usually associated with chloride depletion [8] and it is therefore essential to replace potassium as the chloride salt. Solutions of potassium chloride are unpalatable and the salt is usually given as a capsule or tablet. The administration of simple tablets of potassium chloride, particularly in combination with a benzothiadiazine, has been associated with the development of jejunal ulceration. Recently there have become available in the U.K. two commercial preparations from which the salt is released slowly; these are Slow K (Ciba) and Kloref (Cox-Continental) which contain 600 mg (8 mEq. of potassium) and 500 mg (6·5 mEq. of potassium) of potassium chloride respectively. Usually the patient requires 25–50 mEq. of potassium daily.

CATION EXCHANGE RESINS

These are synthetic polymers which act as weak, insoluble acids and bind cations relatively loosely according to their relative concentrations and the pH of the medium. Generally speaking, they have an affinity in decreasing order for calcium, potassium, sodium and ammonium ions. They are given in a particular phase with the object of removing other cations present in excess.

Ammonium polystyrene sulphonate
Pharmacological actions and therapeutic use. This resin is used in the treatment of resistant oedema. It is usually given orally in a dose of 15 g. three times a day but may be given as an enema in doses of 50–100 g. in 10 per cent dextrose. It is unpalatable and may be partially disguised if given in a flavoured drink or mixed with honey. Sodium ions exchange for ammonium ions and the patient may be spared rigorous dietary sodium restriction.

Contraindications and side effects. The resin may aggravate a severe acidosis and is therefore contraindicated in the presence of renal failure. Potassium ions will be removed along with sodium ions and potassium depletion should be anticipated. This may be overcome with the help of potassium supplements or by giving some of the resin in the potassium phase. Katonium contains 75 per cent ammonium polystyrene sulphonate and 25 per cent potassium polystyrene sulphonate. Minor gastrointestinal disturbances are common.

Sodium polystyrene sulphonate

This resin is used in the treatment of hyperkalaemia in renal failure and is given in the same way as ammonium polystyrene sulphonate. Potassium ions exchange for sodium ions and there is a risk of sodium overload. This has led to the introduction of resin in the calcium phase (calcium polystyrene sulphonate) but hypercalcaemia has been reported after prolonged use and it has been suggested that resin in the aluminium phase is used if prolonged administration becomes necessary.

References

1. Lant, A. F., and Wilson, G. M., *Diuretics in 'Renal Disease'* (1967). Editor Black, D. A. K. Publ. Blackwell Scientific Publications Ltd.
2. Cranston, W. I., Juel-Jansen, B. E., Semmence, A. M., Handfield-Jones, R. P. C., Forbes, J. A., and Mutch, L. M. M., *Lancet* (1963), ii, 966.
3. Dirks, J. H., and Seely, J. F., *Ann. Rev. Pharmacol.* (1969), 9, 73.
4. Fuisz, R. E., *Medicine* (Balt.) (1963), 42, 149.
5. Hutcheon, D. E., Mehta, D., and Romano, A., *Arch. Intern. Med.* (1965), 115, 542.
6. Cannon, P. J., Heinemann, H. O., Stason, W. B., and Laragh, J. H., *Circulation* (1965), 31, 5.
7. Lant, A. F., Smith, A. J., and Wilson, G. M., *Clin. Pharmacol. Ther.* (1969), 10, 50.
8. Schwartz, W. B., de Strihou C. van Y., and Kassirer, J. P., *New Eng. J. Med.* (1968), 279, 630.

This chapter was written by Dr C. S. Ogg (Renal Physician, Guy's Hospital) and edited by Prof. J. R. Trounce.

Category 9

Drugs Used in Haematology

Iron

Iron is commonly administered orally and less often parenterally. Therapeutically, the important consideration is the elemental iron content of the preparation and not simply the total weight of the iron complex in the dose. To achieve a complete response in most cases 1,000–2,000 mg elemental iron must enter the body.

ORAL IRON THERAPY

On average about 20 per cent of the oral dose of an iron preparation is absorbed. Thus to ensure the absorption of 2 g. iron a course of therapy must supply 10 g. iron – the amount of the iron salt used to provide this dose will depend on its iron content. These iron preparations are taken daily and a course should last at least six months.

Ferrous sulphate

Pharmacological action. Haemoglobin biosynthesis.

Therapeutic use. The preferred iron preparation for the treatment of iron–deficiency anaemia. Each tablet contains 200 mg ferrous sulphate of which 60 mg is elemental iron. The usual dose is 1–2 tablets taken three times a day by mouth after meals. For children and those who have difficulty in swallowing tablets liquid preparation in the form of syrups or elixirs are used: 5 ml contains 45 mg elemental iron and the dose is 5–10 ml three times a day after meals. Used prophylactically in pregnancy in a dose of 200 mg daily.

Contraindications and side effects. Like other oral iron preparations, it may irritate the bowel and so exacerbate symptoms in patients with ulcerative colitis or with regional ileitis or in those with a colostomy and is therefore generally contraindicated in these conditions. In some patients oral iron produces nausea and dyspeptic symptoms which can often be avoided or lessened by taking the tablets after meals with a drink of water and by halving the dose. Constipation is not uncommon but if the dose is excessive there may be diarrhoea. Exceptionally an itchy skin rash may develop. All iron preparations blacken the faeces. Patients who are intolerant of ferrous sulphate may do better on either ferrous gluconate or ferrous fumarate or a slow release preparation (see below).

Other iron preparations are only used in those intolerant to ferrous sulphate. Contraindications and side effects are the same as for ferrous sulphate.

Preparation	Elemental iron per tablet	Dose
Ferrous fumarate	65 mg	1–2 tabs t.d.s. after meals
Ferrous gluconate	36 mg	1–2 tabs t.d.s. after meals
Slow Release Preparations		
Ferrogradumet	105 mg	1 tab daily before breakfast
Feospan	45 mg	2–3 caps before meals
Slow Fe	50 mg	1–2 tabs daily

PARENTERAL IRON THERAPY

This form of therapy is reserved for those few patients who fail to respond to adequate doses of oral iron because of intestinal malabsorption or who are intolerant of oral preparations, or for those who are unwilling or cannot be relied on to take tablets regularly for a period of several months. Oral iron should be discontinued at least 48 hours before an injection of iron is given to minimise the danger of generalised reactions.

Iron dextran
Pharmacological action. Haemoglobin biosynthesis.

Therapeutic use. Used intramuscularly usually but can also be given intravenously. 1 ml contains 50 mg elemental iron. Intramuscular injections should be deep and should be confined to the upper outer quadrant of the buttock. A test dose of o·5 ml should be injected first to detect hypersensitivity. Not more than 100 mg (2 ml) should be injected at any one time and to avoid local pain the injection should be made slowly and smoothly. Injections are given at intervals of 1–2 days, alternating the buttocks, until a total dose of 1–2 g. (20–40 ml) has been given. The total dose required can be calculated from the haemoglobin deficit – for every gram of haemoglobin/100 ml in deficit 300 mg iron is given.

Alternatively the total dose of iron dextran can be given as a single intravenous infusion over about 8 hours. The calculated dose of iron-dextran is added to 500 ml normal saline: the infusion rate should not exceed 5–10 drops/minute for the first 30 minutes since reactions will usually be evident in this time and if there is no reaction the infusion rate is increased to 20–30 drops/minute.

Contraindications and side effects. Iron dextran should not be used in patients with a history of allergy or asthma. The skin around the injection site may be stained, sometimes permanently. Intramuscular injections may produce severe local pain if given rapidly. If administered intravenously there may be thrombophlebitis at the infusion site; leakage outside the vein causes intense local pain and an inflammatory reaction follows. Occasional side effects are fever, allergic reactions, enlargement of lymph nodes and arthralgia. Although local sarcomata have been produced in rabbits by the long-term intramuscular injection of large doses of iron dextran there is no evidence that its use in the recommended clinical dosage carries any such risk for man.

Iron-sorbitol

Pharmacological action. Haemoglobin biosynthesis.

Therapeutic use. Used intramuscularly only and the method of administration is similar to that described for iron dextran. About 36 per cent of the injected dose is excreted in the urine and the calculated total dose should be increased by that amount.

Contraindications and side effects. Iron-sorbitol injections may be followed by fever, vomiting, disorientation, a metallic taste and local urticarial reactions. It should not be used if there is a history of allergy or asthma.

Vitamin B_{12}

Pharmacological action. Vitamin B_{12} is an essential co-factor in DNA and protein synthesis and is required for cell division and growth, particularly in rapidly proliferating tissues such as bone marrow and gastrointestinal epithelium. The synthesis and preservation of myelin in nerve tissue is also dependent on an adequate supply of vitamin B_{12}.

Therapeutic use. Used in megaloblastic anaemias due to vitamin B_{12} deficiency: pernicious anaemia, postgastrectomy states, diseases involving the terminal ileum, small intestinal blind loops, infestation with the fish tape worm and in strict vegetarians (vegans). Vitamin B_{12} in the form of hydroxocobalamin is preferred to cyanocobalamin because of better retention and is given by intramuscular injection. For initiating therapy 1,000 μg is given on alternate days for the first week. Thereafter maintenance therapy is essential (except when the cause can be eliminated), and consists of 1,000 μg hydroxocobalamin every two months.

Contraindications and side effects. Vitamin B_{12} should not be used in megaloblastic anaemias due to folic acid deficiency and it is of no value in anaemias not due to vitamin B_{12} deficiency. Very occasionally hypersensitivity reactions may occur.

Folic acid
Pharmacological action. Folic acid is converted in the body into its biologically active form tetrahydrofolic acid by the enzyme folic acid reductase. Its prime roll is to accept and transfer 1-carbon fragments, such as methyl groups, for biosynthesis of purines and thymine and thus of DNA, RNA and proteins. The methyl group is transferred to homocysteine to form methionine and this step requires vitamin B_{12}.

Therapeutic use. It is used in megaloblastic anaemia due to folic acid deficiency. Folic acid is usually administered orally in tablet form. For the treatment of established anaemia a daily dose of 5 mg is given until the blood picture is normal or until the dietary deficiency or malabsorption has been corrected. In pregnancy it is used prophylactically in a daily dose of 400 μg in combination with an iron salt. Folic acid is given by intramuscular injection in a dose of 15 mg if there is vomiting. The reduced form of folic acid, folinic acid, is used to treat toxicity due to folic acid antagonists and a dose of 15 mg is given by intravenous injection.

Contraindications and side effects. Folic acid should not be used in pernicious anaemia. Nor should it be used in other anaemias associated with B_{12} deficiency unless there is also a superadded folic acid deficiency: side effects are almost unknown.

Pyridoxine
Pharmacological action. Pyridoxine is one of the forms of vitamin B_6. It is required for the biosynthesis of haemoglobin. Synthesis of haem is reduced in its absence and consequently utilisation of iron and thus haemoglobin synthesis is impaired.

Therapeutic use. Some cases of congenital and of idiopathic acquired sideroblastic anaemia respond to pyridoxine. It is given by mouth in doses of 500 mg daily and treatment is continued indefinitely. Folic acid deficiency may also be present in such cases if there are associated megaloblastic changes when folic acid and pyridoxine are given together.

ANABOLIC STEROIDS

Methendienone
Pharmacological action. Anabolic steroids increase the sensitivity of erythropoietic stem cells to the action of erythropoietin.

Therapeutic use. Testosterone or a non-virilising anabolic steroid such as methendienone may sometimes stimulate erythropoiesis in hypoplastic anaemia and in myelofibrosis and are worth a trial.

ANTICOAGULANT DRUGS

Heparin
Pharmacological action. In conjunction with a plasma co-factor heparin exerts a direct and immediate anticoagulant effect, both *in vitro* and *in vivo*, by suppressing the activation of prothrombin and inhibiting the action of thrombin. Heparin also has a lipaemia-clearing action via activation of lipoprotein lipase but this effect occurs only *in vivo*.

Therapeutic use. Heparin is used in the prevention and treatment of intravascular thrombosis and embolism, either alone or combined with oral anticoagulant drugs. It cannot be given by mouth since it is destroyed in the gastrointestinal tract and is administered parenterally, usually intravenously. For preventing intravascular coagulation as in cardiac-bypass surgery heparin is used alone in a dose of 300 U/kg and supplemental doses of 150 U/kg are given every 45 minutes during the period of bypass. For treating established thrombosis an initial intravenous dose of 15,000 U is given followed by 10,000 U every 6 hours through an indwelling catheter or needle with a diaphragm. Heparin is also given by continuous infusion: 40,000 U are added to 500 ml saline and infused over 24 hours. Continuous infusion gives a uniform but relatively low level of heparin in the blood and it is important to ascertain that a satisfactory anticoagulant effect is obtained by doing whole blood clotting times on several occasions during the day–the clotting time should be about twice normal. In established thrombosis heparin is usually used in combination with oral anticoagulant drugs which are started at the same time: the heparin is given for 36 hours by which time the oral anticoagulant will have reached a therapeutic level. Heparin has been given by deep subcutaneous injection using a concentrated solution of heparin (25,000 U/ml): a priming intravenous dose of 12,500 units is given followed by 25,000 U subcutaneously every 12 hours. Intramuscular administration is not recommended because of the danger of formation of large painful haematomata.

Contraindications and side effects. Heparin should not be used in the immediate postoperative period because it may cause serious bleeding from the operation site. Otherwise there is little or no danger of serious haemorrhage when the period of heparin administration does not exceed 48 hours. Treatment for longer periods carries a definite risk of haemorrhage which increases with the duration of treatment. Side effects due to hypersensitivity are rare: local wheal formation, erythema, urticaria, macular skin rashes, facial flushing, fever and bronchospasm have been reported. Severe itching and burning of the feet coming on about a week after starting treatment with heparin has also been described. Long-term heparin therapy extending over weeks, although not generally used now has produced alopecia and osteoporosis.

Neutralisation of heparin. This can be rapidly accomplished by giving protamine sulphate intravenously: 1·5 mg, protamine sulphate will neutralise 100 units of heparin. Protamine sulphate is supplied as a solution containing 10 mg/ml and the appropriate volume is injected slowly over a period of 10 minutes. Rapid injection or excessive doses may cause hypotension. If possible the amount of heparin to be neutralised and the effectiveness of neutralisation should be checked by appropriate tests.

ORAL ANTICOAGULANTS

Apart from different dose requirements their pharmacological actions and therapeutic uses are similar and much of what is written about phenindione is applicable to the other preparations as well.

Phenindione

Pharmacological action. Phenindione decreases the coagulability of the blood by depressing the synthesis in the liver of the four vitamin-K dependent plasma clotting factors (prothrombin and factors VII, IX and X). It acts as a competitive inhibitor of vitamin K. With suitable doses of phenindione the plasma concentration of these clotting factors is reduced to the therapeutic level of 5–15 per cent in 36–48 hours. Unlike heparin, phenindione is inactive *in vitro*. It is rapidly and completely absorbed from the bowel within three hours of ingesting the dose. It also has a uricosuric effect.

Therapeutic use. Phenindione is used for the prevention and treatment of thrombosis and embolism. The drug is taken by mouth and dosage is regulated by appropriate tests, usually the prothrombin time test of Quick or the Thrombotest, both tests being carried out on citrated plasma. For safe and effective therapy the prothrombin complex of factors should be maintained between 5 and 15 per cent of the normal level: levels below 5 per cent increase the risk of haemorrhage while levels above 15 per cent are less effective. Very ill patients, those in the early postoperative period or in congestive cardiac failure, those with liver or renal failure and old patients in general, tend to be more sensitive to the anticoagulant action of these drugs than do patients in good general condition. Large and overweight patients usually require higher doses than small and thin patients. The prothrombin time is done before starting treatment. To initiate therapy in patients whose general condition is reasonably good a single dose of 200 mg is given on the first day followed by 100 mg (50 mg b.d.) on the second day. No further doses are given until the results of the 'prothrombin' test, which is done on the third day, is known. The size of subsequent doses for maintenance therapy is dependent on this result: most patients will require a maintenance dose of 50–100 mg daily, given in divided doses in the morning and evening, but some may require doses as high as 175 mg. For patients who may be unduly sensitive the induction doses are halved and daily maintenance doses may be as low as 10 mg: as their general condition improves these patients will require higher doses to keep them in the therapeutic range. If heparin has also been used it is important to ensure that the blood sample for the prothrombin test is taken not less than 8 hours after the cessation of heparin therapy – the presence of heparin will itself prolong the prothrombin time. Some patients can be maintained on a constant daily dose while others are more easily controlled by varying the daily dose, e.g. alternating doses of 50 mg and 75 mg, or a constant dose for 5 days during the week with a lower or higher dose on the remaining days. Tests are done frequently until a stable anticoagulant level has been achieved: thereafter for patients in hospital tests are done once or twice a week, and, for outpatients on long term therapy, once or twice a week for the first two weeks after discharge and then monthly. Patients on long-term treatment should be advised not to vary their diets too much since the amount of vitamin K in the diet will vary with its composition.

Barbiturates and tranquillizing drugs tend to reduce sensitivity to oral anticoagulant drugs. Atromid, phenylbutazone and aspirin tend to increase the sensitivity. In general patients on anticoagulant drugs should not take aspirin or drugs like phenylbutazone.

For elective surgery in patients on long term anticoagulant therapy, the drug is stopped 48 hours before the operation and restarted on the third postoperative day. Postpartum prophylaxis can also be started on the third day.

Contraindications and side effects. Because of the danger of bleeding anticoagulant therapy is potentially dangerous in patients with peptic ulceration or other gastrointestinal lesions which may bleed. Most patients tolerate phenindione very well but a few (1–2 per cent) develop a skin rash which in occasional cases takes the form of a severe exfoliative dermatitis. Haematuria is not uncommon and can usually be brought under control by reducing the dose temporarily. Patients who are otherwise well controlled may develop melaena and this should prompt a search for a local lesion in the gastrointestinal tract. Haemorrhage into the wall of the bowel may give signs of intestinal obstruction and retroperitoneal haemorrhage may lead to ileus. A very occasional side effect of phenindione is agranulocytosis and there are isolated reports of hepatic and of renal damage. Occasional patients develop diarrhoea during phenindione therapy. Drug fever has been reported.

The urine may be coloured pink during phenindione therapy and this should not be mistaken for haematuria.

Intramuscular injections should be avoided in patients on anticoagulant therapy since they may cause painful haematomata.

Warfarin

Pharmacological action. See phenindione. The drug has a longer action than phenindione.

Therapeutic use. See phenindione. For starting treatment a single dose of 40–50 mg is given by mouth. No further doses are given until the third day when the prothrombin time is done. Maintenance doses are usually from 5–10 mg taken as a single dose at about the same time each day. Very ill patients tend to be difficult to stabilise on warfarin but can be controlled more easily with phenindione. For long term therapy, however, warfarin is preferable to phenindione. Warfarin is also used in those patients who have developed hypersensitivity or other reactions to phenindione. Warfarin can be administered intravenously if a patient is vomiting: the intravenous dose is the same as the oral dose. *Contraindications and side effects.* See phenindione. Warfarin appears to cause fewer side effects than phenindione. A few patients may develop nausea, vomiting, or diarrhoea. Occasional patients are completely resistant to the anticoagulant effect of warfarin but they will respond if changed to another drug such as phenindione or nicoumalone.

Nicoumalone (Acenocumarol, *USA*)
Pharmacological action. See phenindione.

Therapeutic use. See phenindione. The drug is administered orally and the induction dose is about 12 mg given in a single dose. Therapeutic levels are reached in 24–48 hours. The results of the prothrombin test on the third day will determine the maintenance dose, which is usually about 4 mg.

Contraindications and side effects. See phenindione. Skin rashes have been reported.

Vitamin K$_1$
Pharmacological action. An essential co-factor in the biosynthesis of four plasma clotting factors: prothrombin, and factors VII, IX and X.

Therapeutic use. An antidote to the action of oral anticoagulant drugs. Used to treat bleeding due to excessive hypoprothrombinaemia. An intravenous dose of 10–20 mg will usually be effective in stopping the bleeding and reducing the prothrombin time in 12–24 hours. Excessive doses should be avoided in patients in whom anticoagulants are to be resumed since they may then be temporarily refractory to treatment. Vitamin K$_1$ is also used in treating the hypoprothrombinaemia associated with obstructive jaundice or severe intestinal-malabsorption – in these cases intravenous doses of 5–10 mg are given.

ε-aminocaproic acid (EACA)
Pharmacological action. EACA is a competitive inhibitor of plasminogen activation.

Therapeutic use. EACA has been used in the treatment of bleeding associated with severe fibrinolysis. Major surgical operations, particularly on the heart and lungs, may be complicated by serious bleeding associated with marked fibrinolysis which leads to digestion of fibrinogen and other clotting factors. In such cases intravenous injection of 5 g. EACA may improve haemostasis but fibrinogen may also have to be administered at the same time if the plasma fibrinogen concentration is below 50 mg/100 ml. Spontaneous bleeding due to fibrinolysis and fibrinogenopaenia occurring in disseminated malignant disease, particularly prostatic carcinoma, may also respond to EACA given either orally or intravenously in a dose of 5 g. which can be repeated for 2–3 doses at intervals of 6 hours. Menorrhagia, in the absence of a local lesion in the uterus, has been reported to respond to oral EACA therapy. EACA has been of value in severe haematuria following prostatic surgery, the dose being 5 g. given orally or intravenously and repeated for not more than 1–2 doses at 6-hourly intervals if necessary.

Contraindications and some side effects. EACA should not be used in chest surgery after closure of the chest since blood clots formed in the pleural or pericardial cavity may be unlysable and then become organised. It should also not be used in bleeding from the upper renal tract because the unlysed clots may lead to permanent obstructive nephropathy. The use of EACA in surgical patients carries the risk of subsequent thrombosis in the postoperative period. EACA is contraindicated in fibrinolysis secondary to disseminated intravascular coagulation.

References
Haematinics

Barkhan, P., *Chapter on Diseases of the Blood in Medical Treatment* (1969), edited by J. MacLean and G. Scott, **II**, p. 281, J. & A. Churchill Ltd., London.

Anticoagulants

Ingram, G. I. C., and Richardson, J., *Anticoagulant Prophylaxis and Treatment* (1965), Charles C. Thomas, Springfield, U.S.A.

Vigran, I. M., *Clinical Anticoagulant Therapy* (1965), Lea and Febiger, Philadelphia, U.S.A.

This chapter was written by Dr P. Barkhan (Consultant Haematologist, Guy's Hospital) and edited by Prof. J. R. Trounce.

Antimicrobials

Benzylpenicillin

Pharmacological action. Like all penicillins benzylpenicillin acts upon dividing bacteria by interfering with cell wall synthesis; it is bactericidal. Inactivated by gastric acid its absorption from the intestine is incomplete. Injected parenterally it is distributed throughout all tissues except bone, nervous tissue and serous spaces. Optimal blood levels are obtained 30–60 minutes after injection, very little being detectable after 6 hours. Sixty per cent is excreted by the kidneys – mainly via the tubules. This route of excretion can be inhibited by probenecid, increasing the blood level for a given dose.

Therapeutic use. Benzylpenicillin is highly effective against infections caused by susceptible organisms principally the Gram-positive cocci (pneumococcus, streptococcus pyogenes, and non-penicillinase producing staphylococcus), Gram-negative cocci (meningococcus and gonococcus), Gram-positive bacilli (clostridia and actinomyces) and Treponema pallidum. Resistance to benzylpenicillin has become a serious problem with penicillinase – producing Staphylococcus aureus.

Ideally it should be given 6-hourly to maintain optimal blood levels. For most infections the dose is 150 mg to 600 mg (250,000–1,000,000 units) intramuscularly every 6 hours until the infection is controlled. In subacute bacterial endocarditis where the organism is less sensitive and relatively inaccessible high doses 6–18 g. daily may be required and this is best given via continuous intravenous infusion. It may be injected into the pleura, pericardium or joints for infections at these sites. Intrathecal injections (not more than 12 mg) have been used in meningitis but inflamed meninges probably allow enough to pass from the blood into the cerebrospinal fluid.

Contraindications and side effects. Benzylpenicillin is virtually free from toxic effects when given intramuscularly in the usual doses although pain at the site of injection is common. Convulsions can follow intrathecal injection and very large intravenous doses in the presence of renal failure may cause encephalopathy. Since benzylpenicillin is supplied either as the sodium or potassium salt, retention of these cations will be important in, for example, bacterial endocarditis or severe renal disease.

The combination of benzylpenicillin with a bacteristatic antibiotic may greatly reduce its efficacy by preventing the former from acting upon dividing bacteria.

Hypersensitivity reactions occur most often in patients with a history of allergy such as eczema and asthma, and when repeated courses of treatment are given. Patients should not, except in extreme illnesses (and then only with suitable precautions), be given penicillin if they have a history of hypersensitivity to it. The common manifestations of this are urticaria, other rashes (including erythema multiforme) and drug fever. Less frequent but more serious effects are wheezing, laryngeal oedema and shock. Others include exfoliative dermatitis, haemolytic anaemia and thrombocytopenia. The Jarisch-Herxheimer reaction should be anticipated in the treatment of tertiary syphilis. Penicillin should not be used topically because of the risk of sensitising the patient and producing resistant organisms.

Procaine penicillin

Pharmacological action. Procaine penicillin differs from benzylpenicillin only by the addition of procaine, thereby slowing absorption and maintaining blood levels for 12–24 hours.

Therapeutic use. It is useful where fewer injections are desired or required on grounds of expediency as in domiciliary practice or in children. The dose is usually 900 mg (1,500,000 Units) once a day or 600 mg (1,000,000 Units) 12-hourly. In order to achieve an optimal blood level quickly it is wise to give with the first injection a dose of benzylpenicillin.

Contraindications and side effects. As for benzylpenicillin. The duration of its effect makes procaine penicillin potentially more dangerous in hypersensitivity reactions. Rare psychotic reactions have been reported after administration of procaine penicillin possibly due to inadvertent intravenous injection.

Phenoxymethylpenicillin

Pharmacological action. Phenoxymethylpenicillin being resistant to gastric acid absorption from the intestine is more reliable and complete than with benzylpenicillin. After absorption the action of the two penicillins is virtually identical although renal excretion is slower.

Therapeutic use. The oral route possesses obvious advantages, particularly in children. For most susceptible infections phenoxymethylpenicillin can be given instead of benzylpenicillin although some clinicians prefer to begin a course of treatment with 'priming' injections of the latter. Tablets are of 125 mg or 250 mg which should be given 6-hourly on an empty stomach. A flavoured oral suspension is available containing 125 mg in 5 ml. Oral penicillin is appropriate in pneumococcal and streptococcal infections of the upper respiratory tract and middle ear. It is also useful in prophylaxis against recurrence of rheumatic fever and glomerulonephritis – the dose being 125 mg or 250 mg daily.

Contraindications and side effects. These are similar to those mentioned for benzylpenicillin although allergy is less frequent. Looseness of the bowels is often encountered and, owing to alteration of the bacterial status quo in the alimentary tract, oral and perineal monilia infection may arise.

Phenethicillin

Phenethicillin is another orally active derivative of 6-amino-penicillinic acid which has no therapeutic advantage over phenoxymethylpenicillin. It is more expensive.

Cloxacillin

Pharmacological action. Cloxacillin is a synthetic penicillin unaffected by penicillinase which is resistant to gastric acid and can therefore be taken by mouth.

Therapeutic use. It is much less active than benzylpenicillin against most organisms except penicillinase producing staphylococci. It should be reserved exclusively for serious systemic infections caused by these organisms which are usually acquired in hospital. It is expensive.

The dose is usually 500 mg every 4 to 6 hours until the infection is under control. It can be given by intramuscular injection when 250 mg 4-6-hourly is usually adequate.

Contraindications and side effects. It is free from direct toxicity. Allergic reactions occur as with other penicillins. Looseness of the bowels and oral or perineal monilia overgrowth are common.

Ampicillin

Pharmacology. Ampicillin is a derivative of 6-amino-penicillinic acid which is resistant to gastric acid and therefore effective by mouth although absorption from the intestine is variable. Sustained blood levels are usually obtained and it is concentrated in the bile and urine. It is rapidly destroyed by penicillinase.

Therapeutic use. Ampicillin differs from other penicillins by being bactericidal to some Gram-negative bacilli including E. coli, some Proteus strains, Salmonellae and Haemophilus influenzae. Urinary tract infections due to susceptible organisms are treated with 500 mg 6-hourly for 10–14 days. In acute exacerbations of chronic bronchitis (frequently associated with Haemophilus influenzae) 500 mg 6-hourly is usually effective, but a very high dose 1 g. 6-hourly for a week reduces the likelihood of subsequent relapse. Typhoid and paratyphoid organisms are very susceptible *in vitro* but infections need to be treated with 1 g. 6-hourly for 14–28 days. Certain coliform organisms produce penicillinase making them resistant to ampicillin.

Contraindications and side effects. Sensitivity rashes are more frequent than with other penicillins and may appear 4–5 days after withdrawal of the drug. Nausea and heartburn are often experienced. Looseness of the bowels may occur and oral and perineal monilia is encountered.

Carbenicillin
Pharmacology. Carbenicillin is a semi-synthetic penicillin active against Ps. aeruginosa and certain Gram-negative organisms including strains of proteus. It is inactivated by penicillinase. Parenteral administration is necessary, high blood and urinary levels are obtained.

Therapeutic use. Carbenicillin may be used in the treatment of severe systemic infections (septicaemia, endocarditis), meningitis and urinary tract infections caused by susceptible organisms which are usually Gram-negative. It may also be used in the treatment or prophylaxis of infection in burns. The intramuscular dose is 1–2 g. 6-hourly but it may be given by slow intravenous injection (3–4 g.) 4-hourly. The dose for children and when renal function is impaired is smaller. Higher blood levels are obtained by the concurrent use of probenecid.

Contraindications and side effects. Pain is common at the site of intramuscular injection and may be relieved by adding a local analgesic. It should not be given to patients known to be hypersensitive to penicillin.

Cephaloridine
Pharmacology. Cephaloridine is a semi-synthetic preparation related to penicillin. Injection is necessary since it is not absorbed from the intestine. After intramuscular injection adequate blood levels are obtained for 8 hours and it is excreted unchanged in the urine.

Therapeutic use. It is highly active against certain streptococci (pneumoniae, pyogenes and viridans) and Staphylococcus aureus even when penicillin resistant. It is also active against E. coli, Proteus mirabilis and some shigella species. The dose is 250 mg or 500 mg 6-hourly for 5–14 days. The intravenous dose is 250 mg. It may be given intrathecally diluting 25 mg in 10 ml of fluid.

Contraindications and side effects. It is not toxic in usual dosage although intrathecally it may cause drowsiness. Skin rashes may occur and caution is required in patients known to be hypersensitive to penicillin since cross sensitivity occurs between these related substances.

Cephalothin is similar to cephaloridine in its action, uses and toxicity.

Cephalexin is a Cephalosporin which is well absorbed from the gut. The oral dose is 0·5–1·0 g. four times daily.

It has a wide anti bacterial activity similar to cephaloridine.

Sodium fusidate

Pharmacology. Sodium fusidate is well absorbed from the intestine and becomes widely distributed in most tissues though not the cerebrospinal fluid. It is active (bactericidal) against penicillinase producing staphylococci.

Therapeutic use. Its use is virtually confined to the treatment of infections due to penicillin resistant staphylococci. Combined with benzylpenicillin it may be more effective but the result is unpredictable. The dose for appropriate infections is 500 mg 3 times daily with or before meals. For children a suspension is available and the dose 23–33 mg/kg daily. Resistance to its action may occur during therapy.

Contraindications and side effects. No serious toxic effects have been reported. Nausea, heartburn and diarrhoea may occur. At present it is extremely expensive.

Tetracyclines

tetracycline	oxytetracycline
chlortetracycline	demethylchlortetracycline
lymecycline	methacycline
chlormethylencycline	tetracycline-phosphate complex.

Pharmacology. The antibacterial activity of the various tetracyclines is virtually identical. They are bacteristatic against a wide range of organisms including most of the pathogenic Gram-negative and Grampositive bacteria (except some strains of proteus and Ps. aeruginosa), certain rickettsiae, large viruses and Entamoeba hystolytica. Absolute cross resistance exists between members of the tetracycline group.

Tetracyclines are usually given by mouth, absorption from the intestine is good and diffusion takes place through most tissues though not well into the cerebrospinal fluid. The liver partly inactivates them by producing protein binding and some metabolic breakdown. Concentration and excretion is high in the bile; the kidneys excrete appreciable amounts.

Good blood levels are obtained for up to 6 hours with tetracycline, oxytetracycline and chlortetracycline. Because of slower excretion demethylchlortetracycline gives adequate blood levels for up to 12 hours.

Therapeutic use. In hospitals there is a growing population of tetracycline resistant organisms, particularly some Gram-negative species and Staphylococcus aureus. Outside hospital the widest use for tetracyclines is in acute exacerbations of chronic bronchitis where the organism is usually either Haemophilus influenzae or Streptococcus pneumoniae. They are the first choice in rickettsial and certain viral infections and the most effective form of therapy for brucellosis. Although effective against E. coli they are not the most appropriate choice for urinary tract infections as they are bacteristatic and resistance often develops.

Tetracycline, oxytetracycline and chlortetracycline are given orally in tablet or capsule form, the dose being 250 mg 6-hourly for most susceptible infections but for more serious ones 500 mg 6-hourly will be necessary. For children a flavoured suspension is available the dose being 30 mg/kg bodyweight daily in divided doses.

The dosage of demethylchlortetracycline is usually 300 mg 12-hourly, methacycline 150 mg 6-hourly and lymecycline 300 mg 6-hourly (100 mg four to six hourly I.M.).

Topical preparations are available for the treatment of skin infections.

Although there are many varieties of tetracyclines the minor differences in absorption and excretion do not offer significant therapeutic advantage.

Contraindications and side effects. Epigastric burning, anorexia, nausea and vomiting are sometimes experienced. Allergy and marrow dyscrasias have been very rarely encountered. Tetracyclines cross the placenta and are deposited in developing bones and teeth of the foetus giving yellow discoloration. They should therefore be avoided in pregnancy and preferably not given to children less than eight years old. Large parenteral doses given in pregnancy have also caused fatal hepatic damage. Infants developing hydrocephalus due to tetracyclines have been reported, and exacerbations of myasthenia gravis may occur when these are given. Renal lesions have followed their use. Phototoxicity is frequent with demethylchlortetracycline and occasionally seen with others.

The most frequent side effects are due to the overgrowth of potentially pathogenic organisms in the alimentary, respiratory and genitourinary tracts. Many patients develop candidiasis of the mouth and gut. In hospital severe staphylococcal infection of the bowel or lung may ensue. Loose stools are commonplace. Pain at the site of injection is relieved by concurrently giving Procaine.

Chloramphenicol

Pharmacology. Chloramphenicol is prepared synthetically. It is well absorbed when given by mouth, readily diffusable into tissues and body fluids including the cerebrospinal fluid. Good blood levels are obtained for up to six hours. It is bacteristatic.

Therapeutic use. The use of chloramphenicol is governed by the fact that it can cause fatal damage to the bone marrow although this is rare. Its range of activity is similar to the tetracyclines but it is particularly effective against salmonellae and other Gram-negative organisms. It is the antibiotic of first choice in typhoid fever when it should be given for 14 days, the dose usually being 500 mg 6-hourly. It is also used in Haemophilus influenzae meningitis in children when it can be given as the succinate parenterally if necessary. It is doubtful if its use can be ustified in other infections except Klebsiella pneumoniae.

Contraindications and side effects. Blood dyscrasias include granulocytopenia, thrombocytopenia and aplastic anaemia. Many fatalities have occurred and are apparently related to the total dose or repeated courses. Circulatory collapse (the 'grey syndrome') causing death may occur in neonates and infants given large doses. Other toxic effects that have been noted are Jarisch-Herxheimer reactions, jaundice, optic neuritis and skin rashes.

Erythromycin

Pharmacology. Several preparations of erythromycin exist which include the base, stearate, ethylcarbonate, estolate which are given orally and the lactobionate which is used parenterally. The range of activity is very similar to that of benzylpenicillin but the erythromycins are usually bacteristatic. The differences between the preparations are mainly in the rate of absorption and the serum levels obtained. The estolate gives somewhat higher and more predictable blood levels and may be bactericidal.

Therapeutic use. With the discovery of newer antibiotics the role of erythromycin has diminished considerably. It is used in common Gram-positive infections in patients known to be allergic to penicillin. Some strains of staphylococci acquired outside hospitals are susceptible but resistance develops rapidly. The dose is 250 or 500 mg 6-hourly depending upon the severity of the infection. Infants and children require 4 to 11 mg per kg 6-hourly. The lactobionate is given by intramuscular injection 2–5 mg per kg three times daily.

Contraindications and side effects. Toxicity is low except with erythromycin estolate which may cause hepatitis and cholestatic jaundice. Heartburn, nausea and looseness of the bowels are common. Acute abdominal pain has been reported. Allergic reactions are uncommon.

Lincomycin

Pharmacology. Lincomycin resembles erythromycin in its properties although chemically it is unrelated. There is evidence that *in vivo* it readily penetrates bone and into the eye.

Therapeutic use. Its ability to penetrate bone makes it useful in the treatment of acute or chronic suppurative osteomyelitis or joint disease caused by penicillin resistant Staphylococcus aureus. It has the advantage that it can be given orally. For acute infections the dose is 500 mg 6-hourly by mouth, the duration of therapy depending on the response. In chronic infections the same dose may be given for 4–6 weeks and then reduced to 8-hourly for as long as a year if necessary.

Contraindications and side effects. Minor gastrointestinal disturbances such as looseness of the bowels are common. Other side effects are few but include skin rashes, granulocytopenia and headache.

Streptomycin

Pharmacology. Streptomycin is bactericidal to certain Gram-negative bacteria and particularly Mycobacterium tuberculosis. It is not absorbed from the intestinal tract and is given therefore by intramuscular injection. Maximum blood level is reached in 1–2 hours and this falls to low levels in about 6 hours. It is distributed in extra cellular fluid (except the CSF) and excreted in the bile and the urine.

Therapeutic use. The principal role of streptomycin is in the treatment of tuberculosis where, to avoid the development of resistant organisms, it is always given in combination with other antituberculous drugs. The usual dose is 1 g. daily I.M., but it may be given 2 or 3 times per week. It may be used in the treatment of urinary tract infections but many organisms are now resistant. It is more effective in alkaline urine. Combined with penicillin in the treatment of Streptococcus viridans endocarcitis synergistic enhancement takes place with improved results. It is useful in the treatment of certain bowel infections namely the dysentery organisms and E. coli. A 5-day course of 1–2 g. daily usually suffices.

Contraindications and side effects. Damage to the inner ear is the most common and serious toxic effect of streptomycin. Both vestibular function and hearing may be involved though the latter is less common. Some individuals are particularly susceptible and the risk is greater in the elderly or patients with impaired renal function. Dihydrostreptomycin is more likely to produce hearing loss. Neuromuscular block leading to respiratory paralysis has been reported following injection of streptomycin into the pleural space.

Skin hypersensitivity reactions are common in persons handling the drug. Allergic reactions by patients are usually of the delayed type (although anaphylactic shock has been reported) manifested as fever, skin rash, arthritis and lymphadenopathy.

Kanamycin

Pharmacology. Kanamycin is similar to streptomycin and neomycin in its antibacterial activity and its pharmacology. Its use is usually confined to parenteral therapy. Peak serum levels are achieved one hour after I.M. injection and it is not detected after six hours. Appreciable quantities are excreted in the urine, very little in the bile.

Therapeutic use. Its main use is in Gram-negative infections. Almost all strains of E. coli and proteus are inhibited by 8 mcg/ml or less *in vitro* and these levels are readily achieved *in vivo*. Many other microorganisms are susceptible but resistance develops rapidly in Staphylococci.

In adults the standard dose is 250 mg I.M. 6-hourly. For children it is 12·5 to 15 mg per kg bodyweight depending on the severity of the infection. Fulminating infections with septicaemia usually require intravenous therapy when the dose is the same as with I.M. injections. It can be given into the peritoneum (250 mg in 500 ml of saline twice daily for 2–3 days) for severe peritoneal infections.

Kanamycin should be reserved for serious infections such as septicaemia resulting from urinary tract infection in pregnancy or the puerperium, proteus septicaemia, E. coli meningitis in the newborn or Gram-negative infections of the peritoneum.

Contraindications and side effects. Ototoxicity occurs particularly in the presence of renal insufficiency when the dose must be reduced. Estimation of the blood concentrations of the drug are useful in these circumstances. Nephrotoxicity in man is relatively low but albuminuria and urinary casts have been reported; tubular damage may occur if therapy is prolonged. Kanamycin shares with streptomycin and neomycin the ability to interfere with neuromuscular transmission particularly after intraperitoneal administration. Allergic reactions are rare.

Neomycin

Pharmacology. Neomycin is closely related to streptomycin and has similar antibacterial activity. Highly toxic parenterally it is used in topical preparations for the eye, ear or skin and may be given by mouth since absorption from the intact intestine is generally low.

Therapeutic use. In tablet form or for children as an elixir it is used for so-called bowel sterilisation before colonic surgery, for the treatment of bacillary dysentery and for certain types of E. coli enteritis. For adults the dose is 500 mg 6-hourly for 5 days for infection and for 3 days pre-operatively. The dose for infants and young children is 50 mg/kg bodyweight daily divided into four doses.

Numerous topical preparations are available for use in infections of the conjunctivae, external ear and skin. It is combined with bacitracin and polymixin in aerosols or fine powders for wounds or operation sites.

Contraindications and side effects. The high degree of ototoxicity precludes its use parenterally. Neomycin may damage the intestinal mucosa causing malabsorption. While usually hardly any of the drug is absorbed, in certain circumstances this may be important. Kidney damage has been reported after oral use. It shares with streptomycin a curare-like action enhanced by the use of muscle relaxants and certain types of general anaesthesia. Topical use of neomycin has led to an increasing incidence of skin hypersensitivity.

Gentamycin

Pharmacology. Gentamycin is related to streptomycin chemically and in its range of action against Gram-negative organisms. It is also effective against Ps. aeruginosa. It is given by intramuscular injection and excreted by the kidneys.

Therapeutic use. Its use has been largely confined to urinary tract infections by susceptible organisms. Serious systemic infections have been successfully treated. The dose is 0·8–1·2 mg/kg daily given in 3 equal doses 8-hourly.

Contraindications and side effects. The main toxic effects are upon the inner ear and labyrinthine damage is more frequent when renal function is impaired. Hypersensitivity has so far been uncommon.

Polymixin B

Pharmacology. Polymixin B is poorly absorbed from the alimentary tract and is therefore given parenterally when it is excreted in the urine. It is also used topically for ophthalmic and skin infections.

Therapeutic use. Polymixin B is active against Ps. aeruginosa and other Gram-negative organisms but is used when resistance to safer antibiotics has been demonstrated. Infections of the urinary tract or meningitis due to Ps. aeruginosa are the situations where it is most useful. The dosage is 50 mg (500,000 Units) 8-hourly by intramuscular injection combined with procaine to relieve local pain. It is effective topically in the treatment of infected burns and otitis externa where it is often combined with bacitracin.

Contraindications and side effects. Topical therapy is safe and hypersensitivity uncommon. Parenterally it is toxic to the kidneys and neurological disturbances (paraesthesiae, neuromuscular block, convulsions) have been reported.

Colistin

Pharmacology. Colistin which is identical to polymixin E is very similar in its pharmacological properties to polymixin B.

Therapeutic use. The indications for the use of colistin are the same as those for polymixin B, namely infections (particularly of the urinary tract) due to Ps. aeruginosa. The preparation for injection is called Colistin Sulphomethate and in the USA this is combined with a local analgesic. The dosage is usually 1,000,000 Units 8 hourly.

Contraindications and side effects. These are similar to those with polymixin B.

Sulphonamides

Pharmacology. Although there are numerous sulphonamide preparations with different properties certain generalisations can be made. Some are insoluble and when taken orally remain within the intestine but most are readily absorbed from the gastro-intestinal tract. After absorption there is variable protein binding, acetylation and excretion by the kidney. The rate of excretion and the degree of penetration into the cerebrospinal fluid are related to the amount of protein binding. Their action is to inhibit folic acid synthesis of bacteria by competing with its precursor para-aminobenzoic acid to which they are chemically related. This action is bacteriostatic.

Therapeutic use. Sulphonamides are active against Gram-positive and Gram-negative cocci and certain Gram-negative bacilli. They are inhibited by the presence of pus. Clinically they are most useful in treatment of infections of the urinary tract and meningococcal meningitis (although resistant meningococci have been reported in the USA). Formerly used in bacillary dysentery they are now less useful as resistant strains are common. Occasionally a particular sulphonamide may be useful in bacterial conjunctivitis, trachoma, toxoplasmosis, nocardiosis and dermatitis herpetiformis.

For systemic infections sulphadiazine or sulphadimide are used most often with a loading dose of 3–6 g. followed by 1–2 g. 4- or 6-hourly. For children a quarter or half this dosage applies. These preparations can be used for urinary tract infections, half the above adult dose is then adequate.

Other sulphonamides are used in urinary tract infections such as sulphamethizole (0·2 g. then 0·1 g. 4-hourly) or sulphafurazole. The choice is wide but the effects of the various preparations is similar. The long acting sulphonamides include sulphamethoxypyridazine and sulphadimethoxine the dosage of these being 1 g. daily.

Sulphonamides are sometimes used parenterally in the treatment of bacterial meningitis particularly in the UK when sulphadiazine is usually chosen. Other soluble sulphonamides are equally effective. These are best given via an intravenous saline infusion since it is important to ensure adequate hydration. The dose is usually 6 g. per 24 hours.

Contraindications and side effects. Numerous adverse effects have been described and the reported incidence varies between 1 and 15 per cent. Hypersensitivity reactions are fairly common and include fever and a variety of mild or serious skin eruptions. Almost all types of haematological disorders can occur. Gastrointestinal disturbances are usually minor but are very common; jaundice may be encountered. Crystalluria may occur if the urine is acid and concentrated. Other effects include arteritis and certain neurological disturbances.

Trimethoprim

Pharmacology. Trimethoprim has a similar range of action to the sulphonamides. It inhibits the enzyme which reduces dihydrofolic acid to tetrahydrofolic acid – a stage in purine synthesis which follows that arrested by sulphonamides. The combination of trimethroprim with a sulphonamide produces a synergistic action which is much more effective than either substance alone. Trimethoprim is well absorbed after oral administration. It is slowly excreted by the kidney and adequate blood levels are obtained by 12-hourly doses. It penetrates to the cerebrospinal fluid.

It is available in combination with sulphamethoxazole, each tablet containing 80 mg Trimethoprim and 400 mg of the sulphonamide.

Therapeutic use. The combination of trimethoprim and sulphamethoxazole is active against most of the pyogenic cocci (but have no advantage over the penicillins in this respect) and many Gram-negative organisms. The principal use is in infections of the urinary tract and for acute exacerbations of chronic bronchitis. The dose is usually two tablets twice daily. Gonorrhoea has also been effectively treated. The scope of this combination has not yet been fully discovered.

Contraindications and toxic effects. Toxic effects have so far been rare but leucopenia has been reported. Trimethoprim should not be given early in pregnancy as teratogenic effects have been observed in experimental animals.

Isoniazid

Pharmacology. Isoniazid (Isonicotinic acid hydrazide, INAH) is a synthetic substance very active against Mycobacterium tuberculosis. It is well absorbed after an oral dose and is distributed throughout body fluids including cerebrospinal fluid. The ability to acetylate (inactivate) the drug is genetically determined and varies considerably between racial groups.

Therapeutic use. Isoniazid is only used in the treatment of all forms of tuberculosis but since resistance develops if it is used alone it should always be used in combination with at least one other antituberculous drug – usually PAS. The usual dosage is 300 mg daily in two or three doses. It is presented in many forms either alone or in combination with PAS. It can be given intramuscularly and intrathecally but these routes are rarely required.

Contraindications and toxic effects. The incidence of side effects is low but allergic reactions have occasionally been reported. The most important toxic effect is peripheral neuropathy which is commonest among slow inactivators. Rare adverse reactions include jaundice, psychosis, endocrine disturbances and a lupus erythematosus-like syndrome.

Para-aminosalicylic acid (PAS)

Pharmacology. PAS is usually administered as the sodium or calcium salt. It is active against Mycobacterium tuberculosis although less so than streptomycin or INAH. It is well absorbed from the alimentary tract and distributed throughout body fluids but with poor penetration into the cerebrospinal fluid. Excretion via the kidneys is rapid.

Therapeutic use. Its use is confined to the treatment of tuberculosis always in combination with at least one other drug since resistance develops if it is used alone. Many preparations are available in tablet, powder or granular form usually in combination with INAH. The daily dose should ideally be 20 g. but in practice 12 g. is usually the maximum that is tolerated. It should be given with food. The main purpose of combining PAS with INAH is to ensure that patients take both (or neither) to mitigate the risk of resistance developing to one drug alone.

Contraindications and side effects. Nausea, anorexia, and abdominal discomfort are common. Diarrhoea may occur. Hypersensitivity in the form of fever, skin rashes and lymphadenopathy are encountered. Desensitisation is often possible. Other reactions include pulmonary infiltration with eosinophilia, goitre with hypothyroidism, jaundice and haematological abnormalities.

Rifampicin

Pharmacology. Rifampicin is a new antibiotic active against Gram-positive bacteria and some Gram-negative bacteria as well as Mycobacterium tuberculosis where its activity is similar to that of isoniazid. It is well absorbed by the oral route and readily diffusable into the tissues. It is mainly excreted in the bile.

Therapeutic use. The role of rifampicin has not yet been defined but it is useful in the treatment of tuberculosis. At present it should be used only when organisms are resistant to first line drugs. The dose is 450–600 mg daily as a single dose. It should be given in combination with at least one other drug to prevent emergence of resistant strains.

Contraindications and side effects. Toxicity in man has not yet been fully studied but hepatic function may be impaired. Eosinophilia and leucopenia have been reported. Nausea occurs occasionally. It causes red discoloration of the sputum and urine. Patients with hepatic disease should not be treated with rifampicin and until further information is available it should be avoided in pregnancy.

Pyrazinamide
Pharmacology. Pyrazanamide is very active against mycobacterium tuberculosis. It is well absorbed when taken orally, and diffuses into the body fluids. It is excreted by the kidneys.

Therapeutic use. Pyrazinamide is a second line drug for the treatment ot tuberculosis. The dosage is 30 mg per kg bodyweight daily in four doses, but this should not exceed 3 g. per day.

Contraindications and side effects. Liver damage is common and may be fatal. Estimations of the serum transaminases should accompany its use. It may precipitate gout and cause skin rashes.

Ethionamide
Pharmacology. Ethionamide is chemically related to INAH but not as effective. Absorption by mouth is good and distribution takes place throughout body fluids including the cerebrospinal fluid.

Therapeutic use. Ethionamide is used in the treatment of tuberculosis when organisms are resistant to the safer and more effective drugs. The dose is 0·5 g. twice daily.

Contraindications and side effects. Side effects are common and include vomiting, diarrhoea, peripheral neuropathy, convulsions and hepatic damage.

Cycloserine
Pharmacology. Cycloserine is well absorbed from the intestine and freely diffusable throughout tissue fluids including the cerebrospinal fluid. It is excreted by the kidneys.

Therapeutic use. It is used as a second line drug in the treatment of tuberculosis. The dosage is 1 g. daily in two doses but therapy should begin with 250 mg twice daily, increasing slowly by increments of 250 mg each week.

Contraindications and side effects. Serious toxic effects are relatively common and include psychoses, depression and convulsions.

Ethambutol

Pharmacology. Ethambutol is well absorbed by the oral route and excretion is predominantly via the kidney.

Therapeutic use. This is a relatively new second line antituberculous drug. The dose is usually 25 mg per kg bodyweight daily.

Contraindications and side effects. The most important toxic effect of ethambutol is optic neuritis producing diminished visual acuity and central scotoma. Patients should have complete ophthalmological examination before therapy and visual acuity should be checked regularly during treatment. Other effects include rare instances of gastrointestinal disturbance and allergy.

Nalidixic acid

Pharmacology. Nalidixic acid, a synthetic preparation, is well absorbed after oral administration and largely excreted (80 per cent) in the urine where it appears in high concentrations.

Therapeutic use. The role of nalidixic acid is confined to the treatment of urinary tract infections where it is effective against many Gram-negative organisms. It must be used in high dosage (at least 4 g. per day) but resistance frequently occurs during therapy. Successful treatment is less likely in the presence of abnormalities of the urinary tract and deep seated infections of the kidney respond poorly.

Contraindications and side effects. Adverse effects are few and mild but include allergic reactions (rashes, fever) haemolytic anaemia, skin photosensitivity, respiratory depression, a variety of disturbances in the nervous system and occasional nausea or vomiting. It causes positive reactions in the urine to 'Clinitest'.

Nitrofurantoin

Pharmacology. Nitrofurantoin is a synthetic preparation which is absorbed from the gut and excreted in high concentration in the urine. Excretion is enhanced if the urine is acid. Blood levels are low at the usual dosage. It is effective against a large number of Gram-negative and Gram-positive organisms.

Therapeutic use. Its use is confined to the treatment of infections of the urinary tract by susceptible organisms. It is often useful against E. coli and some proteus infections. The dose for adults is 100 mg 6-hourly after food or, for prophylaxis, 50 mg 12-hourly. In renal failure its efficacy is reduced since less is excreted.

Contraindications and side effects. Nausea and vomiting occur frequently. Pulmonary infiltration and asthma have been reported. Nitrofurantoin has caused megaloblastic anaemia, and haemolytic anaemia – particularly in glucose-6-phosphate dehydrogenase deficiency. Peripheral neuropathy has been encountered, chiefly where there is impaired renal function.

Amphotericin B

Pharmacology. Amphotericin B is poorly absorbed from the alimentary tract. It is given by intravenous infusion. Urinary excretion is slow and adequate blood levels persist for long periods.

Therapeutic use. It is the drug of choice in systemic fungal disease and is indicated in serious infections due to candidiasis, histoplasmosis, coccidioidomycosis, cryptococcosis and blastomycosis. The dose is 1·0 mg/kg daily given by infusion over a period of 6 hours. The duration of therapy depends on severity of the infection and the response but it may be necessary to continue for several weeks.

Amphotericin B is available in tablet (10 mg) form for the treatment of oral candida infection.

For fungal meningitis 0·5 mg mixed with 20 mg of hydrocortisone can be given intrathecally.

Contraindications and side effects. Kidney damage occurs in nearly all patients given amphotericin B intravenously. The renal lesion, which may be permanent, consists of tubular swelling with calcification. Fever, nausea, vomiting, anorexia and severe malaise are common. They are to some extent mitigated by giving 50 mg hydrocortisone at the start of each infusion. Nearly all patients develop a normocytic normochromic anaemia. Intrathecal injection often produces severe headache.

Nystatin

Pharmacology. Nystatin is an antifungal antibiotic which is poorly absorbed from the alimentary tract.

Therapeutic use. It is used principally in the treatment of infections by Candida albicans. Lesions in the mouth respond to 500,000 units in the suspension given 8-hourly. Monilial vaginitis is treated with pessaries (100,000 units) inserted once or twice daily. Candidiasis of the intestine is treated by tablets or the suspension. It may be given as an aerosol or inhaled in powder form for pulmonary candidiasis and aspergillosis.

Contraindications and side effects. Toxicity is low and side effects are few. It has an unpleasant taste and nausea, vomiting and diarrhoea occasionally occur.

Griseofulvin

Pharmacology. Griseofulvin is partly but adequately absorbed from the alimentary tract and is then selectively taken up by precursors of keratin. It is particularly effective against superficial fungal infections of the hair, nails and skin.

Therapeutic use. It is the treatment of choice in ringworm of the nails and hair. Treatment is usually necessary for weeks or months since new keratin, free from the fungus, may be reinfected by the old keratin before this has been shed.

Dosage for adults is 0·5 g. daily either as one or two doses. Children require 125 to 250 mg daily. The course of therapy should be continued until after the fungus has disappeared from scrapings of previously infected tissue.

Contraindications and side effects. Nausea and abdominal discomfort are occasionally experienced. Depression of the white count has been reported and griseofulvin antagonises the action warfarin. Skin rashes and, rarely, photosensitivity may occur. Other infrequent adverse effects include allergic reactions, transient proteinuria, mood change, gynaecomastia in children and disturbances in porphyrin metabolism. The drug should be avoided in porphyria.

This chapter was written by Dr R. K. Knight (Physician, Guy's Hospital) and edited by Prof. J. R. Trounce.

Category II

Drugs Used in Tropical Medicine

THE TREATMENT OF AMOEBIASIS

Dehydroemetine hydrochloride

Pharmacological action. This drug is lethal to the parasites in the tissue phase of amoebic infection. It does not affect the organisms in the intestine.

Therapeutic use [1]. The daily dose is 60 mg given intramuscularly; for children the daily dosage is calculated as 1 mg/kg of bodyweight. Treatment is given daily for up to 10 days. Because of the cardiotoxic effect of the drug the patient is kept in bed during the treatment, and he should avoid strenuous activity for a further three or four weeks. At least two weeks must elapse between courses if administration is repeated.

Side effects and contraindications. 1. Local pain and sterile abscess formation may result from tissue necrosis. A fresh site should be chosen for each injection.

2. The drug has a direct toxic action on the myocardium. Tachycardia, a fall of blood pressure and the development of a gallop rhythm may occur. Electrocardiographic changes consisting of T-wave change, prolongation of the PR interval, widening of the QRS complexes, and alterations in rhythm may be noted. The drug should be stopped if there is evidence of heart block.

3. Nausea and vomiting may be produced.

4. Toxic effect on skeletal muscle. Pain, tenderness and stiffness may occur in the muscles of the legs, arm and neck.

Contraindications. Heart disease, particularly if there is danger of heart failure or arrhythmia; pregnancy, due to toxic effect on the foetus; polyneuritis of recent development.

Emetine bismuth iodide
Pharmacological action. This is a derivative of emetine which is administered orally and, being only partially absorbed, it acts in the in-

testinal lumen as well as in the intestinal wall. It has a direct lethal effect on the organisms.

Therapeutic use [1]. The dose is 60 mg three times a day; it often produces considerable nausea, so that it should be given at night. Phenobarbitone or some other antiemetic preparation may be required.

The effect in the tissues is slow and rather weak so that ideally a 10-day course by mouth should be preceded by treatment with emetine by injection for 3 or 4 days.

The patient's activity should be strictly restricted but confinement to bed is not necessary. The pulse rate and blood pressure should be recorded daily. Unusual changes call for electrocardiography.

Side effects and contraindications. The drug is liable to cause nausea and vomiting; it is therefore prescribed in gelatin capsules or as enteric-coated tablets to lessen these side effects; an antiemetic may also be used.

Chloroquine

Pharmacological action. This drug is effective against the extra-intestinal phase of the infection, and is indicated when it is considered that the parasite has extended beyond the intestinal lumen. Its particular value is in the treatment of hepatic amoebiasis.

Therapeutic use. 150 mg of chloroquine base twice daily for 20 days.

Side effects. See section on malaria.

Diiodohydroxyquinolone (diiodoquin)

Pharmacological action. This is an intraluminal amoebicide and is essential if re-invasion of the tissues is to be avoided and if the patient's stools are to be rendered non-infectious. This drug is one of many intraluminal amoebicides; it is not the only effective one, but it is the best established.

Therapeutic use. 600 mg three times daily for 20 days, given orally.

Side effects and contraindications. The drug is usually free from unpleasant side effects; rarely it may produce mild iodism. The drug should not be given if there is a history of idiosyncrasy to iodine.

Metronidazole

Pharmacological action. This is an imidazole compound which has amoebicidal properties. It is active against amoebae in the liver as well as in the bowel. This is its advantage over most of the other amoebicidal drugs.

Therapeutic use. 800 mg three times a day orally for 10 days.

Side effects and contraindications. The drug is relatively non-toxic. Nausea occurs in some cases.

THE TREATMENT OF VISCERAL LEISHMANIASIS (syn. Kala-azar)

Pentavalent compounds of antimony

Pharmacological action. The mode of action of these compounds is not certain; they probably inhibit essential enzymes in the parasite by reacting with free thiol groups. Pentavalent antimony is rapidly excreted, principally via the kidneys.

Therapeutic use [2]. (a) **Sodium stibogluconate (Solustibosan)** is the most widely used preparation and is also the least toxic. It is issued in ampoules of sterile isotonic neutral solution in water so that 1 ml contains 20 mg of antimony. It can be given intramuscularly or intravenously. The initial dose is 6 ml for sensitivity test. Thereafter it is given in the dose of 15 mg/kg of bodyweight intravenously or intramuscularly for from 10 to 30 days. On account of the danger of allergic reactions it is advised that a break of ten days should be made between the fifth and sixth injections, if any untoward symptoms have been observed. To effect a cure this course of treatment may have to be repeated after an interval of a month.

(b) **Urea-stibamine.** This preparation is undoubtedly efficient and often succeeds where other pentavalent salts fail. In resistant cases it may be given in combination with neostibosan. The total amount to effect a cure is about 3 g. intramuscularly or intravenously in doses of 100 to 200 mg on alternate days for about one month; if, for some reason or other, intermission in treatment takes place, the parasites tend to become antimony-fast.

(c) **Ethylstibamine (neostibosan)**

Side effects and contraindications. Sodium stibogluconate is virtually free from side effects. However, all antimonials can produce a metallic taste in the mouth and throat, and mild gastrointestinal symptoms such as vomiting, diarrhoea and abdominal discomfort. These symptoms are uncommon.

Urea-stibamine may rarely give rise to such symptoms as an urticarial rash, a sense of suffocation following each injection, and collapse due to an anaphylactic reaction.

THE TREATMENT OF TRYPANOSOMIASIS

Suramin

Pharmacological action. This drug is effective against both Trypanosoma gambiense and Trypanosoma rhodesiense present in the blood and in the lymph nodes. The drug does not cross the blood-brain barrier. Suramin-resistant strains do not occur, so that this drug is given as first choice.

Therapeutic use. The drug is used for the early stage of trypanosomiasis, before there are signs of central nervous system involvement and with a normal cerebrospinal fluid. The adult dose is 1 g. intravenously each week for five weeks. Each injection is freshly prepared prior to administration. A test dose of 0·2 g. is given intravenously at the onset of treatment; if there is no untoward effect the patient is given 0·8 g. on the following day. For patients weighing less than 50 kg the weekly dose can be calculated as 20 mg/kg of bodyweight.

Side effects and contraindications. These include idiosyncrasy, with collapse after injection, renal damage with proteinuria, skin rash, conjunctivitis, stomatitis, hypotension, peripheral neuropathy and bone marrow depression. The drug is contraindicated in renal disease or in adrenal insufficiency.

Pentamidine

Pharmacological action. The pharmacological action and indications for use of this drug are much the same as for suramin. However, the development of pentamidine-resistant strains of Trypanosomes has been noted in East Africa. Like suramin, pentamidine does not cross the blood-brain barrier.

Therapeutic use. A course of treatment consists of 10 daily injections intramuscularly of 4 mg/kg of bodyweight. The solution must be freshly made. Local tissue reaction may occur at the site of injection; for this reason care must be taken to select a fresh site for each injection. (Some clinicians prefer the intravenous route.)

Side effects and contraindications. These are unusual and may occur irrespective of the route by which the injections are given, viz. faintness, hypotension, bradycardia, vertigo, sweating, salivation, nausea, vomiting, diarrhoea, epigastric discomfort, pruritus and urticaria.

Intravenous injections may cause syncope associated with a sudden fall in blood pressure, and there may be dyspnoea and constricting pain in the chest.

Tryparsamide

Pharmacological action. This drug is a pentavalent arsenical which is able to cross the blood-brain barrier and has consequently been used for many years for cases of trypanosomiasis with signs of involvement of the central nervous system and/or with an abnormal cerebrospinal fluid.

Side effects and contraindications. There are several disadvantages to its use:

(a) it has numerous serious toxic effects; notably optic neuritis and dermatitis;

(b) it is ineffective against T. rhodesiense infections;

(c) T. gambiense is becoming increasingly resistant to the drug;

(d) to be effective it needs to be given in combination with suramin.

On this account its place has largely been taken by melarsoprol.

Melarsoprol (Mel. B)

Pharmacological action. This drug is a combination of a trivalent arsenical with dimercaprol (BAL). It has the capacity of penetrating the blood-brain barrier and is given for cerebral forms of the disease. Both T. rhodesiense and T. gambiense respond. A 90 per cent cure rate and 5 per cent relapse rate has been reported with this drug.

Therapeutic use [3]. Some physicians have found the drug uncomfortably toxic and special care is advocated in its administration.

(a) For mild invasion of the nervous system three injections of 3·6 mg per kg of bodyweight to a maximum of 200 mg are given intravenously on alternate days.

(b) If the nervous system is seriously affected, two courses (as above) are given at an interval of three weeks.

(c) Relapses should be treated with a repeat course.

Side effects and contraindications. (a) Minor side effects include headache, abdominal discomfort, colic, vomiting, diarrhoea, urticarial rash, pyrexial reactions of the Herxheimer type.

(b) Exfoliative dermatitis.

(c) Toxic hepatitis.

(d) Arsenical encephalopathy.

Treatment of serious side effects should be by withdrawing the drug and giving a course of dimercaprol (BAL) as soon as possible.

THE TREATMENT OF LEPROSY

Damino-diphenysulphone (dapsone, DDS)

Pharmacological action. This is the parent drug of the sulphone group. It is effective, but cure even in favourable cases is slow. It is recognised as being the drug of choice, though some patients show intolerance. However, there are indications that resistance to dapsone may appear in leprosy bacilli (the number of cases in which this has been demonstrated is still small), and there is a possibility of relapse in lepromatous leprosy.

Therapeutic use. Dapsone is given in gradually increasing doses; for adults, 25 mg twice a week or 10 mg daily for 6 days each week (200 mg twice a week may be enough, especially in field work). For children the doses must be correspondingly lowered. Treatment should be taken regularly for 2–4 years.

Side effects. Most toxic reactions occur during the initial weeks of treatment.

1. Generalised dermatitis – patients can be desensitised by giving very small and gradually increasing doses.

2. Erythema nodosum leprosum, an allergic reaction sometimes seen in lepromatous or dimorphous leprosy, may be precipitated. Treatment of this form of leprous reaction requires experience. Corticosteroids may be necessary.

THE TREATMENT OF BILHARZIASIS
(syn. Schistosomiasis, bilharzia)

Niridazole (Ambilhar)

Pharmacological action. This drug is effective against S. haematobium, S. Mansoni and S. japonicum.

Therapeutic use. It is administered orally. Dosage is 25 mg/kg of body-weight daily in two or three divided doses for 7–10 days. Tablets of 500 mg are available for adults, and of 100 mg for children. Maximum adult daily dosage is 2 g./day.

The drug is equally effective in urinary and intestinal bilharziasis. In urinary bilharziasis and mild intestinal infections the patient need not be confined to bed during the course of treatment, and may continue at work or at school. However, in the presence of hepato-splenic bilharziasis patients should be confined to bed because of the risk of neuro-psychiatric disturbance.

Side effects and contraindications. Side effects are usually mild. They are more likely to occur in adults than in children. The minor toxic effects are gastrointestinal irritation and tachycardia. Neuropsychiatric disturbances have been recorded in patients with heavy intestinal infections; these include episodic excitement, euphoria, hallucinations, disorientation, generalised convulsions, localised muscle tremors and spasms. The urine takes on a cola-colour during treatment. ECG and EEG changes have been described.

Niridazole is incompatible with isoniazid (INH).

Sodium antimony tartrate

Pharmacological action. The pharmacological actions of antimony are in general similar to those of arsenic. This drug affects schistosomes by interfering with a glycolytic enzyme in the parasite. It affects all forms of schistosomiasis.

Therapeutic use [4]. A course consists of twelve intravenous injections on alternate days. Each injection is given in 10 ml of saline and the solution must be freshly prepared. The initial dose is 30 mg, the second 60 mg, the third 90 mg; subsequently 120 mg may be given. The full dose for children is 2 mg per kg of bodyweight. The injection should be given slowly.

Side effects and contraindications. 1. The drug is a tissue irritant and must be given intravenously; great care should be taken to ensure it is not injected outside a vein.

2. Gastrointestinal irritation may be produced.

3. Cough is thought to be due to minute emboli to the lungs; rarely pulmonary oedema and pneumonia have complicated its use.

4. The drug is a cardiac depressant; bradycardia and even severe hypotension may follow its use, so that the patient should lie down during the injection and for one hour subsequently.

5. Occasionally exfoliative dermatitis may occur. This is an indication for Dimercaprol therapy. Herpes zoster occurs quite commonly with the intensive use of antimony.

The drug is contraindicated in febrile patients and in cases of cardiac, respiratory, renal or hepatic disease.

Lucanthone (Miracil D)

Pharmacological action. This drug has a limited field of use in the treatment of bilharziasis (S. haematobium infection), for it is not as successful in curing S. mansoni infection. A cure rate of about 60 per cent may be anticipated.

Therapeutic use [5]. A daily adult dose of 1–2 g. in two divided doses is given for three consecutive days (children 25 mg per kg bodyweight daily).

Side effects. Nausea and mental depression may be produced. The skin and tongue may become yellow and the palms and soles reddish brown in colour.

Caution should be used in patients with impaired renal function.

ANTHELMINTICS

Hydroxychlorobenzamide (Niclosamide, *USA*)
Pharmacological action. The drug is a derivative of salicylamide.

Therapeutic use. The drug has eclipsed all older methods in the treatment of taeniasis. It is effective against the beef tapeworm (Taenia saginata), the pork tapeworm (Taenia solium) and the fish tapeworm (Diphyllobothrium latum).

On waking in the morning two tablets of 0·5 g. are chewed thoroughly and swallowed with a little water. One hour later this is repeated. There is no need for fasting or purgation. Two hours after the last dose a light breakfast can be taken, and the patient can eat normally thereafter. Children under 4 years require half a tablet at each dose, and those between 4 and 8 years require 1 tablet.

In the unlikely event of failure, the drug can be given the following time for two days instead of one, i.e. a total of 8 tablets.

Piperazine
Pharmacological action. The drug is highly effective against both Ascaris lumbricoides and Enterobius vermicularis. The effects of piperazine on ascaris have been investigated extensively. The gross effect of the drug on the ascaris is a paralysis of muscle that results in expulsion of the

worm by peristalsis. The drug has been shown to block the response to acetylcholine of ascaris muscle. Orally administered piperazine is well absorbed but it is almost devoid of pharmacological activity in the host.

Therapeutic use. The official preparation is piperazine citrate. In ascariasis a single daily dose of 3·5 g. is given for two consecutive days; this is the maximum dose. Children should be treated with 75 mg/kg. This dosage will cure almost 100 per cent of patients. In oxyuriasis, single daily doses of 65 mg/kg with a maximum of 2·5 g. given for 8 days will result in 95–100 per cent cure.

It is unnecessary to supplement treatment with cathartics or enemas. Prior fasting is not necessary.

Side effects. Very occasionally gastrointestinal upset, transient neurological effects, and urticarial reactions have attended its use.

Piperazine has been used without ill effect during pregnancy. There are no contraindications to its use.

Thiobendazole

Pharmacological action. This drug is effective in hookworm, roundworm (ascaris), threadworm and whipworm infestations. The drug has specific anthelminthic activity.

Therapeutic use. Given as an emulsion or as chewable tablets of 500 mg; the dosage is 25 mg/kg of bodyweight twice daily for 2 days. The emulsion is put up in bottles of 15 ml and for an adult weighing over 60 kg, the dose is 7·5 ml twice daily for 2 days. The drug should be taken immediately after food to reduce gastric irritation. No purgation is required.

Side effects and contraindications. These are mild but common, and occur in about one-third of patients; they include dizziness, anorexia, nausea, vomiting, diarrhoea, headache, visual disturbance. There are no contraindications to its use.

Bephenium

Pharmacological action. The drug is very effective against Ascaris lumbricoides and hookworms, and moderately effective against whipworms. Very little of the drug is absorbed. It is of particular value in mixed ascaris and hookworm infestation.

Therapeutic use. The drug should be taken on an empty stomach, and food may be taken one hour later. The dose is 5 g. for adults or children; half of this dose for infants.

Side effects. Nausea, vomiting, diarrhoea, dizziness and headache may occur.

Diethyl carbamazine

Pharmacological action. The drug is used in the treatment of filariasis. It removes the microfilariae of Wucheraria bancrofti rapidly, but its action on the adult worms is less certain. In onchocerca infection caused by the filarial worm – Onchocerca volvulus – the microfilariae are killed but the adult worms survive. In sandworm disease (larva migrans) it is effective. Good results have been obtained in cases of tropical eosinophilia.

Therapeutic use. In Wucheraria bancrofti infestation 150–500 mg is given daily; for Onchocerca volvulus the dose is 2 mg per kg once on the first day, twice on the second day, then thrice daily for 30 days. In tropical eosinophilia the drug is given three times a day for five days.

Side effects. Headache, anorexia, nausea and vomiting occur in some patients. The release of proteins from the death of the worms in the tissues can produce allergic reactions.

THE TREATMENT OF MALARIA

Chloroquine

Pharmacological action. The drug has the ability to enter the red blood cells in high concentration, and to exert a schizonticidal effect in malaria. It persists for a long time in the body and is therefore effective in long-term suppression of malarial infection. It is effective against all four species of human malarial parasites.

Therapeutic use [5]. 1. Treatment of acute primary attacks of malaria in non-immune subjects. An initial loading dose of 600 mg is given, followed by a 300 mg dose six hours later, and 300 mg on each of the next two days. Smaller doses may suffice to treat relapses and to treat immune subjects.

2. In the chemoprophylaxis of malaria, either given alone or in combination with primaquine. Dose is 0·5 g. of chloroquine phosphate, given on the same day of each week.

3. For cerebral malaria, chloroquine (the equivalent of 200–300 mg base) by intravenous or intramuscular injection, repeated in four hours and then followed by oral administration as above.

Side effects and contraindications. Toxic side effects are rare. Minor side effects such as headache, blurred vision, pruritus, gastrointestinal distress and restlessness have been reported. Serious, irreversible retinal damage is an extremely rare complication of chloroquine therapy when it is given for malaria. The drug is contraindicated in pregnancy as it crosses the placenta and it has caused neurological damage in the foetus.

Quinacrine

Pharmacological action. This drug is effective against the asexual parasites in their erythrocytic phase.

Therapeutic use [6]. If chloroquine or other 4-amino-quinolines are not available, quinacrine is the drug recommended for use.

1. For an acute attack 200 mg are given every three or four hours, five times on day one, followed by 100 mg three times a day for the next six days.

2. For prophylaxis or suppressive treatment 100 mg of quinacrine is given daily; this should begin two weeks before exposure and continue for at least four weeks after exposure.

Side effects and contraindications. Side effects are chiefly cutaneous, gastrointestinal and neurological. Various types of dermatitis; yellow cutaneous and conjunctival discoloration, abdominal distress, nausea, vomiting and diarrhoea have been reported. In rare instances toxic psychosis has occurred.

Quinine

Pharmacological action. The drug is effective against asexual parasites in the erythrocytic phase. However, it passes into the red cell from the plasma with some difficulty, so that high doses are required for it to be effective. It is rapidly metabolised by the body and excreted, so that six- to eight-hourly dosage is necessary to maintain effective drug levels in the plasma.

Therapeutic use [6]. Acute attacks of malaria in non-immune subjects may be treated by the administration of 600 mg of quinine sulphate every eight hours for five to seven days. Radical cure of infections with certain strains of P. falciparum may require the daily administration of 2 g. of quinine for seven to ten days.

In serious cases of malignant tertian malaria, e.g. in coma, quinine is given intravenously as quinine dihydrochloride 300–600 mg well diluted in 100–200 ml sterile normal saline and injected very slowly (thirty minutes)

With quinine the risk of the parasite developing drug resistance is not great.

Side effects and contraindications. Symptoms of cinchonism are frequent – headache, nausea, vomiting, ringing in the ears, diminished auditory acuity, blurred vision and giddiness. These symptoms usually subside rapidly after cessation of treatment, but permanent auditory or visual damage have occurred in rare instances. The existence of a causal relationship between quinine and haemoglobinuric (blackwater) fever has not been proved. Rapid intravenous injection may precipitate cardiac failure.

Pregnancy is a contraindication to its use.

Primaquine

Pharmacological action. The drug is mainly effective against pre-erythrocytic schizonts and gametocytes. It is less effective against erythrocytic parasites. It is quickly degraded and eliminated by the body.

Therapeutic use. For prophylaxis of malaria 45 mg of primaquine base is given weekly together with 300 mg of chloroquine base. This regimen has been particularly successful against vivax and malarial malarias, but it is less successful in preventing overt falciparum malaria. For the radical cure of relapsing P. vivax malaria the equivalent of 15 mg of primaquine base is given daily for 14 days.

Side effects and contraindications. Acute haemolytic anaemia may develop in patients whose red cells are deficient in the enzyme glucose-6-phosphate dehydrogenase (G–6–PD). This enzyme deficiency is genetic, but the exact mechanism of the haemolysis is not known. This haemolytic anaemia is often considerably more severe in Caucasians than in Negroes.

The drug should not be given together with quinacrine or sulphadiazine which enhance its toxic effects.

Proguanil

Pharmacological action. The action of this drug is slow as it acts in the body only after being changed to an active metabolite. It is effective against both erythrocytic and exoerythrocytic parasites; its fundamental action is to inhibit the nuclear division in the developing schizont.

Therapeutic use. For suppressive purposes the dose for adults is 100–300 mg daily.

Side effects and contraindications. Proguanil is practically non-toxic. Large doses may cause vomiting. Prolonged use causes loss of appetite, weight and energy.

Pyrimethamine

Pharmacological action. This drug has schizonticidal activity. It is an antimetabolite of folic acid; it may in this way inhibit the nuclear division of the developing schizont.

Therapeutic use [5]. As a suppressant of malaria with prolonged action, 25–50 mg weekly. Its action is too slow for it to be recommended for treatment of an acute attack of malaria.

Side effects and contraindications. Pyrimethamine may produce leuco-penia and thrombocytopenia. Megoloblastic anaemia has been des-cribed. The rapid development of drug resistance has been reported.

References

1. Wilmot, A. J., *Clinical Amoebiasis* (1962), Oxford, Blackwell.
2. Manson-Bahr, P., *Manson's Tropical Diseases* (1966), 125, Baillière, Tindall and Cassell, London.
3. WHO Expert Committee on Trypanosomiasis, 1962.
4. Maclean, K., and Scott, G., *Medical Treatment* (1969), 458, Churchill, London.
5. Sapeika, N., *Actions and uses of Drugs* (1966), 171, Balkema, Cape Town.
6. Berberian, D. A., *Amer. J. Med.* (1969), **46**, 96.

This chapter was written by Dr P. I. Folb (Dept of Clinical Pharmacology, Guy's Hospital) and edited by Prof. J. R. Trounce.

Category 12

Cytotoxic Drugs

THE ALKYLATING AGENTS

These compounds have the general formula:

$$R—CH_2CH_2^+$$

They are capable of combining with a number of chemical groupings found in the cell. These include thiols, carboxyl, phosphate, amino and nucleic acid groups. Their effect on tumours is probably due to their linking with guanine in the DNA chain. It seems that cross linkage between the DNA strands by alkylating agents is of particular importance. Alkylating agents thus interfere with mitosis and they may also produce abnormalities of the chromosomes.

The various alkylating agents, although having the same general action differ considerably in their solubility, absorption, penetration and speed of action. It also seems that certain alkylating agents are particularly effective in certain types of tumour; the reason for this is not known.

All this group of drugs damage normal cells, particularly those of the bone marrow and intestinal tract, and this is one of the main limitations of their use.

NITROGEN MUSTARDS

Mustine (Mechlorethamine, USA)

Pharmacological action. Mustine is a highly reactive alkylating agent. It is rapidly transformed in solution into an ethyleneimmonium ion which is the active alkylating agent *in vivo*. Mustine is a highly irritant substance and can therefore only be given intravenously. After injection it rapidly combines with various groups and is cleared from the blood within a few minutes.

Therapeutic use. Mustine must be freshly made up before administration: it rapidly combines with water in solution. It is important to avoid extravasation of the drug around the vein and it is safest to set up an intravenous infusion of 5 per cent dextrose and to inject the dose of mustine through the tubing with the drip running rapidly.

Mustine often causes nausea and vomiting for some hours after administration. The patient will suffer less upset if it is given in the evening combined with chlorpromazine 25–50 mg I.M. and a hypnotic.

The usual total dose of mustine is 0·4 mg/kg. It can be given as a single injection, or the course can be spread over several injections – usually 0·1 mg/kg on alternate days for four injections. Larger doses have been used but this causes a considerable increase in side effects [1]. Mustine produces a rapid response in those with susceptible tumours.

Mustine can also be given intrapleurally or intraperitoneally in patients with recurrent malignant effusions. The usual dose is 20 mg as a single injection and the volume of the effusion should be reduced if possible to around 500 ml to produce optimal results. Little systemic absorption occurs and bone marrow depression is rare. Mustine may cause a temporary increase in the effusion but it should be effective within three weeks; if not it can be repeated.

Neoplasms which usually respond well to mustine are:

Hodgkin's disease
Lymphosarcoma
Reticulum celled sarcoma

Neoplasms which sometimes show response to mustine are:

Carcinoma of the bronchus
Carcinoma of the ovary
Carcinoma of the breast
Seminomas.

Side effects and contraindications. Depression of the bone marrow is the most important toxic action of the drug. It affects the granulocytes and sometimes the platelets, and rarely it also causes erythrocyte depression. These effects are maximal about 10–14 days after giving the drug and they may clear up in 3–4 weeks.

Mustine usually produces severe nausea and vomiting (see above) and may also cause diarrhoea and even ulceration of the gut. Rarely it causes rashes.

Great care must be taken if mustine is given to those with existing bone marrow depression. If it is essential to give the drug, a considerably smaller dose should be used and the bone marrow examined regularly. Facilities should also be available to nurse patients with severe leukopoenia.

Mustine should also be avoided (as should all cytotoxic agents) in the first three months of pregnancy. Although evidence from human sources is scanty, there is good experimental evidence that it can cause foetal abnormalities.

Degranol

Degranol is a mannitol–mustine compound. It is given intravenously and does not appear to have advantages over mustine.

Chlorambucil

Pharmacological action. Chlorambucil is a mustine–phenylbutyric acid compound. It is relatively non-irritant and is satisfactorily absorbed after oral administration.

Therapeutic use. The usual dose is 0·1–0·2 mg/kg daily as a single dose in the morning. It is usually two or three weeks before a response is seen and the course of treatment lasts three to five weeks. This may be followed by maintenance treatment at a dose of 2·0 mg daily.

   Neoplasms which respond well to chlorambucil are:
      Chronic lymphatic leukaemia
      Hodgkin's disease and reticulum–celled sarcoma
   Neoplasms which occasionally respond to chlorambucil are:
      Carcinomas of the ovary and testicles.
Because of its predominant action on the lymphocyte series of cells chlorambucil has also been used as an immunosuppressive agent, and in the treatment of macroglobulinaemia.

Side effects and contraindications. Bone marrow depression can occur especially if the bone marrow is depressed or infiltrated. Weekly white counts are therefore required. Nausea occurs in about 10 per cent of patients and it can rarely cause rashes.

Cyclophosphamide

Pharmacological action. Cyclophosphamide is inactive *in vitro*; in the body it is split by the enzyme phosphoramidase, liberating an alkylating agent. It was originally hoped that this would occur predominantly in tumours, but it is now realised that activation occurs throughout the body. It is well absorbed from the intestine and partially excreted in the urine where it may set up a chemical cystitis.

Therapeutic uses [4]. The dose of cyclophosphamide is between 3–6 mg/kg daily and it can be given orally or intravenously. The high dose level should not be continued for more than five days and this may be followed by an oral maintenance dose of 2·0 mg/kg per day.

Neoplasms which often respond well to cyclophosphamide are:
Hodgkin's disease and other lymphomas
Multiple myeloma
Burkitt's tumour*
Maintenance therapy in acute lymphoblastic leukaemia.
Neoplasms which may show some response are:
Carcinoma of the breast and ovary
Neuroblastomas.

Cyclophosphamide in doses of around 100 mg per day can also be used as an immunosuppressive.

Side effects and contraindications. Cyclophosphamide will produce leukopoenia and regular white counts are required. However, it rarely causes platelet depression. About a third of the patients develop some degree of alopecia which is reversible. A few patients develop a chemical cystitis with haematuria and a high fluid intake is advisable. Other side effects include rashes and nausea.

Melphalan

Pharmacological action. Melphalan is a compound of phenylalanine and mustine. It was hoped that the combination of mustine with a naturally occurring substance would increase its activity. It is well absorbed from the intestinal tract. It differs from mustine in that after absorption it remains active for several hours.

Therapeutic uses. Melphalan is largely used in treating multiple myelomatosis [5]. It has also been used with some success in seminomas and ovarian carcinomas and in treating melanomas by local perfusion, about half the patients showing some response. The usual dose is 5–8 mg daily for 10 days. When the bone marrow has recovered this may be followed by a maintenance dose of 1–2 mg daily.

Side effects and contraindications. Melphalan is a powerful depressive of the bone marrow, producing leukopoenia, and in particular, platelet depression. It may also cause nausea and with large courses some degree of alopoecia.

THE ALKYL SULPHONATES

Busulphan

Pharmacological action. Busulphan is well absorbed from the intestine. It appears to react particularly with thiol groups and the major portion is excreted as sulphur-containing metabolites.

* Africans appear to tolerate cyclophosphamide very well and large doses are given (30 mg/kg for 5 days).

It depresses the myeloid series of cells and has much less effect on the lymphocytes.

Therapeutic uses. Busulphan is used in chronic myeloid leukaemia where it nearly always produces remission. It is also occasionally used in polycythaemia rubra vera. It is the drug of choice for treating thrombocythaemia.

The initial dose is between 3·0–6·0 mg daily. This is continued until the total white count reaches 20,000/cu.m.m. The drug is then stopped and the white cell count usually continues to fall for 2–3 weeks.

If the white cell count then rises rapidly a continuous maintenance dose of busulphan is required; usually 2·0 mg daily, with the object of keeping the white count at about 10,000 per cu.m.m. If the white count only rises slowly further treatment is delayed until the white count rises to about 50,000 cu m.m. or troublesome symptoms develop. Intermittent courses are used in such cases. Blood counts are done at 2–4 week intervals.

Side effects and contraindications. Depression of the myeloid of cells has already been discussed, and it is important to remember that it is occasionally irreversible and may also affect the platelets. Pigmentation of the skin is quite common with prolonged treatment and is thought to be due to a disturbance of tyrosine metabolism.

A few patients complain of weakness, nausea and hypotension, reminiscent of adrenal failure – but adrenal function is normal.

Diffuse interstitial pulmonary fibrosis has been reported; its cause is unknown.

Mannitol myleran
Mannitol myleran is given orally but nausea is common. Its uses are similar to those of mustine and it has no particular advantages.

THE ETHYLENAMINES

Triethylene melamine
Triethylene melamine has been used in lymphomas. However its absorption is variable, and therefore the therapeutic dose varies between patients, and sometimes severe toxic effects may be produced. It is rarely used at the present time.

ThioTEPA
ThioTEPA is given by intramuscular or intravenous injection as it is rapidly hydrolysed in the stomach when given orally.

It appears most effective in carcinomas of the ovary and breast, and it has been suggested that this is due to depression of endocrine function rather than a direct action on the tumour.

ThioTEPA can be given:

1st week:	10 mg daily for 5 days
2nd week:	10 mg daily for 4 days
3rd week:	10 mg daily for 3 days
Thereafter	2 mg weekly.

ThioTEPA produces bone marrow depression in a very arbitory manner and as it has little advantage over other alkylating agents, it is now rarely used.

ANTIMETABOLITES

These drugs resemble substances used by cells for their metabolism and growth.

They compete with the normal substrates of cell metabolism and thus may prevent cell growth and ultimately cause cell death.

The action of antimetabolites is not confined to malignant cells but they are useful in certain types of malignant disease, probably because they have their greatest effect on rapidly dividing cells. Ultimately their usefulness is limited by their toxicity to normal cells, particularly those of the bone marrow, or to the development of resistance.

FOLIC ACID ANTAGONISTS

Methotrexate

Pharmacological action. Methotrexate competes with folic acid for the enzyme dihydrofolic reductase. It has a very much greater affinity for the enzyme than folic acid and thus effectively blocks the synthesis of tetrahydrofolic acid, an important substance in the synthesis of purines.

This block can be circumvented by giving folinic acid, which is 5 fumerzl-tetrahydrofolic acid, a stage further on in purine synthesis.

About half a normal dose is absorbed and largely excreted unchanged in the urine within forty-eight hours. Only a small quantity penetrates the blood-brain barrier (see below).

Therapeutic uses. Methotrexate will produce a remission in about 50 per cent of children with acute leukaemia. It is also used for maintenance treatment when a remission has been induced by other drugs. It is best used for maintenance rather than induction of a remission in acute lymphoblastic leukaemia.

To induce a remission the dose is 2·5–5·0 mg daily in children, and 2·5–10·0 mg daily in adults. Although methotrexate can be given by injection it is usually given orally as a single dose on an empty stomach. This is important, as multiple doses during the day may not produce the same effect. This regime is continued for 3–4 weeks, until a remission is induced or toxic effects appear.

There are a variety of schemes for maintenance treatment. One method is to give 20 mg/m² of body surface twice weekly.

Methotrexate can also be used in meningeal leukaemia. It is given intrathecally in doses of 0·2 mg/kg on alternate days for a total of four doses, and this should be combined with folinic acid 5·0 mg I.M. to reduce systemic effects.

Methotrexate is also used with considerable success in the treatment of chorionepithelioma [6]. Higher doses are used and treatment requires special facilities.

Side effects and contraindications. In addition to bone marrow depression methotrexate causes oral ulceration which is preceded by patches of hyperaemia. It may also cause nausea, diarrhoea and alopecia.

Methotrexate should be used with care in patients with impaired renal function, as a high proportion of the drug is excreted via the kidneys.

PYRAMIDINE ANTAGONISTS

5-Fluorouracil

Pharmacological action. This drug interferes with the synthesis of nucleic acid. It is poorly absorbed after oral administration, and is usually given intravenously. Most of the drug is metabolised, and about 20 per cent is excreted in the urine.

Therapeutic uses. 5-Fluorouracil is of some benefit in about 30 per cent of patients with carcinoma of the ovary, stomach, intestinal tract and breast [7].

The usual dose is 15 mg/kg*/day for 5 days – the daily dose should not exceed 1·0 g. If there is no sign of toxicity a further four doses of 7·5 mg/kg can be given on alternate days.

Side effects and contraindications. Early signs of toxicity are nausea, anorexia and diarrhoea. If mouth ulceration develops the drug should be stopped.

Bone marrow depression is common and usually starts within a few

* This is ideal body weight.

days of starting treatment. Reduced dosage should be used in those with bone marrow depression or jaundice.

5-Fluorouracil is contraindicated in patients who have had an adrenalectomy as they are particularly sensitive to the diarrhoea and vomiting produced by this drug.

PURINE ANALOGUES

6-Mercaptopurine

Pharmacological action 6-Mercaptopurine interferes with the synthesis of DNA.

The essential stage is probably the conversion of 6-mercaptopurine to its ribose phosphate derivative which either prevents DNA synthesis or leads to the formation of abnormal DNA.

6-Mercaptopurine is well absorbed and widely distributed in the body. However, penetration into the CSF is poor. It is rapidly metabolised and the metabolites are excreted in the urine.

Therapeutic uses. 6-mercaptopurine is used in treating acute leukaemia, producing a remission in about 30 per cent of children and a smaller proportion of adults. The dose is 2·5 mg/kg daily by mouth and is given as a single dose. The initial course should not exceed six weeks and is continued until a remission is produced or toxic effects appear. It is usually used in combination with other drugs in producing a remission. 6-mercaptopurine can be used for maintenance therapy, the usual dose being 1·0 mg/kg daily.

6-mercaptopurine in combination with other cytotoxic agents is used in treating chorionic carcinoma.

Side effects and contraindications. In addition to bone marrow depression 6-mercaptopurine occasionally causes nausea, vomiting and diarrhoea. Jaundice, which can be either cholestatic or due to cellular damage, has been reported.

The concurrent use of allopurinol with 6-mercaptopurine increases the toxicity of 6-mercaptopurine and the dose should then be halved.

Azathioprine

Pharmacology and therapeutic uses. Azathioprine is a 6-mercaptopurine derivative. It has been widely used to suppress rejection of transplanted organs and in the treatment of diseases (nephrotic syndrome, systemic lupus, and some types of haemolytic anaemia) which are believed to have an autoimmune basis. It is given orally in doses of 2–4 mg/kg bodyweight. Azathioprine can cause bone marrow depression with leucopenia and more rarely thrombocytopoenia. It is therefore desirable in patients on this drug to have white cell and platelet counts at regular intervals.

PLANT PRODUCTS

Vinca alkaloids

A number of alkaloids have been isolated from the periwinkle and two of them, *vinblastine* and *vincristine*, have been shown to have useful cytotoxic action.

Pharmacological action. Both of these alkaloids inhibit cell division at the metaphase but this does not appear to be their chief mode of antitumour action.

They are poorly absorbed from the intestine and are usually given intravenously.

They are rapidly excreted by the liver and therefore any biliary obstruction will increase the effect of the drug.

Therapeutic uses. **Vinblastine** is used in treating Hodgkin's disease, and chorionepithelioma.

The initial dose is 0·1 mg/kg intravenously; this is increased by 0·05 mg/kg each dose being given at weekly intervals until a remission is produced or toxicity occurs. Weekly dosage should not exceed 0·3 mg/kg. Maintenance treatment can be given weekly at a dose level which is found by trial not to produce leucopenia. A blood count should be performed before each dose.

Side effects and contraindications. Vinblastine can cause depression of the bone marrow. It usually occurs within a week of the dose, and is short lived.

Vincristine is used as the initial drug in treating acute leukaemia. It can also be used in Hodgkin's disease and related conditions; it is particularly useful when there is bone marrow infiltration as it has little depressing effect on leucocyte or platelet formation. The initial dose is 0·01 mg/kg intravenously; this is increased by 0·01 mg/kg given at weekly intervals until a remission is produced or toxicity appears.

Side effects and contraindications. The toxic effects of vincristine are mainly on the nervous system. Muscle weakness effects, particularly the dorsiflexors of the feet, the hands and larynx. This is followed by loss of reflexes and paraesthesiae. The autonomic nervous system is also affected, causing constipation and signs suggesting intestinal obstruction. Nerve damage usually recovers if the drug is stopped, but may persist indefinitely.

Vincristine also produces some alopecia. Depression of the bone marrow can occur but is usually preceded by neurotoxicity.

ANTIBIOTICS

Several antibiotics have been found to have antitumour activity.

Actinomycins probably produce their effect by interference with DNA and protein synthesis.

Actinomycin D (Dactinomycin, *USA*) is used in the treatment of Wilms' tumour in association with surgery and radiotherapy. It is given intravenously in doses of 15 micrograms/kg body weight daily for 5 days.

Toxic effects include dryness of skin, nausea, vomiting and bone marrow depression.

Actinomycin C can be used in Hodgkin's disease in doses of 200 μg daily until a total of 1·5 mg has been given.

Rubidomycin (Daunomycin, *USA*) is used in producing rapid remission in acute leukaemia. It is given intravenously in doses of 1·0 mg/kg daily for 3–4 days.

Toxic effects include rapidly developing marrow depression (daily white counts are required), nausea, vomiting and ulceration of the mouth. Heart failure is produced by large doses.

MISCELLANEOUS COMPOUNDS

Procarbazine (Methylhydrazine, *USA*)
Pharmacology and therapeutic uses. Procarbazine is most useful in Hodgkin's disease when it induces a remission in about 60 per cent of patients. It may also produce some benefit in reticulum-celled sarcoma. Its mode of action is unknown. The initial dose is 50 mg daily orally, and this can be increased to 200 mg daily. A course usually lasts three weeks unless the white count or platelets become depressed.

Procarbazine can be used for maintenance treatment in doses of 100 mg daily.

It can also be given intravenously but this is rarely necessary.

Side effects and contraindications. Procarbazine depresses the bone marrow. In addition it may produce nausea and vomiting. It is an amine oxidase inhibitor and potentiates phenothiazine which should therefore be used in half the normal dose if given concurrently.

Hormones. Oestrogens and steroids are used in various neoplastic conditions.

References
1. Weisberger, A. S., *Ann. N.Y. Acad. Sci.* (1958), **68**, 1097.
2. Ezdwill, E. Z., and Schutzman, L., *J. Amer. med Ass.* (1965), **191**, 444.
3. Galton, D. G., Wiltshaw, E., Szur, L., and Dacie, J. V., *Brit. J. Haemat.* (1961), **7**, 73.
4. Hamilton Fairley, G., and Simester, J. M., Editor *Cyclophosphamide (Endoxance)* (1964), J. Wright, Bristol.
5. Galton, D. G., and Peto, R., *Brit. J. Haemat.* (1968), **15**, 331.
6. Bagshawe, K. D., *Brit. med. J.* (1963), **2**, 1303.
7. Ansfield, F. J., Schroeder, J. M., and Currer, A. L., *J. Amer. med. Ass.* (1962), **181**, 295.
8. Boesen, E. G., Davis, W., *Cytotoxic Drugs in the Treatment of Cancer* (1969), Edward Arnold Ltd, London.

This chapter was written by Prof. J. R. Trounce.

Category 13

Drugs Used in the Treatment of Hormonal Disorders

PITUITARY HORMONES

Growth hormone
This is only available in small amounts for the treatment of hypopituitary dwarfism.

Gonadotrophins

Preparations	Source
Chorionic gonadotrophin injection.	Extract of pregnancy urine.
Human follicle stimulating hormone.	Extract of post-menopausal urine.

Therapeutic uses. Female infertility [1]. An accurate diagnosis is essential before treatment is begun, because primary ovarian failure and mechanical causes are not amenable to treatment with gonadotrophins. The essence of treatment is the initial treatment with FSH injection to induce maturation of the follicle, followed by the administration of HCG to induce ovulation. There are many different treatment regimes, but the treatment must always be monitored carefully with one or more of the following serial measurements: urinary oestrogens, vaginal smears, basal body temperatures and pregnanediol.

Male infertility. This is less well established than female infertility, but successful results have been reported in patients with hypopituitarism and some types of testicular abnormalities.

Undescended testes and delayed puberty. HCG in doses of 1,000–2,000 units, two to three times weekly in six weekly courses are commonly used, but the exact indications and optimum ages are controversial.

Side effects. Allergic reactions may occur.

Hyperstimulation syndrome during the treatment of female infertility with ovarion enlargement abdominal pain and even ascites and pleural effusion.

Clomiphene

Preparation. Clomiphene citrate tablets, 50 g.

Pharmacology. Clomiphene is a non-steroid compound related to the oestrogen chlorotrianisene. It has weak oestrogenic properties but its principle property is the ability to cause increased secretion of gonadotrophins by the pituitary. Clomiphene may exert this effect by blocking the inhibitory effect of other oestrogens on the hypothalamus.

Therapeutic uses [2]. Clomiphene citrate is used for the treatment of infertility due to disorders of ovulation. It is ineffective, however, in cases of complete pituitary or ovarian failure. The usual dose is 50 mg daily for five days; if this induces ovulation then the course is repeated until a pregnancy occurs. If not, then the dose is increased to 100 mg daily for five to ten days.

Side effects. Hot flushes due to the increased level of gonadotrophin are frequent; ovarian enlargement occurs, but with careful supervision the incidence can be reduced. Headache, diplopia, dizziness, transient scotomata, constipation, allergic skin reactions, and reversible hair loss have been reported and there is a higher incidence of multiple pregnancy.

Thyroid stimulating hormone

Preparation. Thyrotrophin injection.

Therapeutic uses. TSH, in conjunction with radioiodine uptake measurements is used diagnostically to differentiate between primary and secondary hypothyroidism, to diagnose myxoedema in patients already receiving thyroid medication, and also to confirm hypothyroidism when the results of radioiodine investigations are borderline. It is sometimes used to increase the uptake of a therapeutic dose of radioiodine in the treatment of functioning thyroid carcinomas.

The dose is 2.5 to 10 units I.M. daily.

Vasopressin

Pharmacology. Apart from its effect on smooth muscle causing a rise in arterial blood pressure and other manifestations of smooth muscle contraction, vasopressin is also the antidiuretic hormone increasing the permeability of the collecting ducts of the kidneys to water and thereby producing a hypertonic urine.

Side effects and contraindications. Vasoconstriction leads to skin pallor and a rise in arterial blood pressure.

Smooth muscle contraction may cause nausea, intestinal cramp and uterine contractions.

Constriction of the coronary vessels may occur and therefore should not be given if there is evidence of coronary artery disease.

Posterior pituitary snuff may cause local allergic reactions with nasal congestion, and allergic pulmonary infiltration has been described.

Preparation	Main use	Dose
Vasopressin injection	Diagnosis of diabetes insipidus	0·1 unit I.V.
	Treatment of bleeding oesophageal varices	20 units in I.V. infusion in 10 mins.
Vasopressin tannate injection	Diagnosis and treatment of diabetes insipidus	2·5–5 units I.M.
Lypressin injection*	Diagnosis of pituitary-adrenal insufficiency	10 units I.M.
Lypressin nasal spray*	Treatment of diabetes insipidus	10 units 3–6 times daily
Pituitary (posterior lobe) insufflation	Treatment of diabetes insipidus	5–20 mg t.d.s.

* Synthetic preparations.

Thyroid hormones

Preparations	Equivalent doses
Thyroid extract tablets	30 mg
U.K. Thyroxine sodium BP (Sodium levothyroxine, USA)	0·05 mg
Sodium liothyronine	10 μg.

Pharmacology. The main action of the thyroid hormones is to uncouple oxidative phosphorylation in mitochondria, but they undoubtedly also stimulate a large number of other enzyme activities.

The principle difference between thyroxine and liothyronine is in the duration of action; thyroxine has a peak action occurring at nine days and lasting for about eighteen days, whereas liothyronine has a peak action at two to three days and lasts for only eight days.

Therapeutic uses. Thyroxine is used in the treatment of primary or secondary hypothyroidism. The starting dose should be low (0·025–

0·05 mg daily) and gradually increased at fortnightly intervals to a full replacement dose of 0·2–0·4 mg daily. Thyroxine is also used in the treatment of simple goitres, acute and chronic thyroiditis, and has been used in suppressive doses in the treatment of functioning thyroid carcinomas.

Liothyronine is used in the treatment of myxoedema coma; the dose is 25 μg every six hours.

Side effects. Excessive dosage is characterised by many of the features of thyrotoxicosis, in particular tachycardia, nervousness, tremor and sweating. During the initial stages of the treatment of myxoedema, there may be precipitation of coronary insufficiency, cerebrovascular disease or failure of the pituitary adrenal axis.

ANTITHYROID DRUGS [3]

Thiocarbamides

UK and USA	Initial dose	Maintenance dose
Methimazole	10 mg (5–20) 8–hourly	5–10 mg daily
Carbimazole	15 mg (5–20) 8–hourly	5–20 mg daily
Methylthiouracil	150 mg (100–200) b.d.	50–150 mg daily
Propylthiouracil	200 mg (100–300) b.d.	50–200 mg daily

Pharmacology. The thiocarbamides act by inhibiting the oxidation of iodide to iodine, and interfere with the coupling of iodotyrosines in the production of triiodothyronine and thyroxine. They are rapidly absorbed by the gastrointestinal tract and excreted in the urine. They also cross the placenta and are excreted in breast milk.

Therapeutic uses. They are used to treat thyrotoxicosis, either as the primary treatment or in preparation for thyroidectomy. The initial dose is high until the patient is euthyroid (three to six weeks). Thereafter a smaller maintenance dose is required.

Side effects and contraindications. Skin rashes which may be associated with arthralgia and lymphadenopathy. Mild gastrointestinal upsets, leucopenia, agranulocytosis (which is usually reversible) have been reported.

The incidence of side effects is lowest with methimazole and propylthiouracil.

These drugs should be used with caution if there is tracheal compression, and in thyrotoxicosis associated with pregnancy.

Other antithyroid drugs

Potassium perchlorate acts by competitive inhibition of the thyroidal iodine concentrating mechanism, and also releases any unbound intrathyroid iodine.

Therapeutic uses. In view of the unacceptable toxicity in therapeutic doses, it is only used for diagnostic purposes: 600 mg of perchlorate will discharge radioiodine from the thyroid affected by some forms of dyshormonogenesis.

Side effects include nephrotic syndrome, aplastic anaemia, neutropenia skin rashes, pancytopenia, gastrointestinal upsets.

Iodine

Preparations. Aqueous iodine solution (Lugols) 5 per cent iodine, 10 per cent potassium iodide.

Iodobrassid tablets (USA) containing 293 mg iodine.

Pharmacology. Iodine in thyrotoxicosis arrests the cellular hyperplasia, increases the storage of colloid and decreases the release of thyroxine. The vascularity of the gland is diminished. The maximum effect of iodine occurs at about ten days, but is only maintained for two to three weeks, in spite of continued administration.

Therapeutic use. After preparation for surgery with one of the thiocarbamide group of drugs, iodine may be used for ten to fourteen days preoperatively to diminish the vascularity of the gland. The dose is 0·3–1 ml of aqueous iodine solution daily in milk. Larger doses are used in the treatment of thyrotoxic crises (2–3 ml daily).

Side effects. Gastric irritation and rarely there is hypersensitivity to iodine with fever and skin rashes.

DRUGS AFFECTING CALCIUM METABOLISM

Parathyroid hormone

Preparation. Parathyroid injection (containing 100 units/ml).

Pharmacology. Parathyroid hormone increases calcium absorption from the gut, increases calcium resorption from bone, and decreases renal excretion of calcium. It also increases the renal excretion of phosphate. The peak effect of one injection occurs at about eighteen hours and lasts for up to thirty-six hours.

Therapeutic use. The only use is in the acute treatment of hypoparathyroid tetany. The initial dose is 100–300 units I.M. or S.C., followed by 20–100 units hourly, depending on the serum calcium level. Prolonged treatment is associated with the development of tolerance.

Side effects. Hypercalcaemia, and allergic reactions.

Vitamin D
Preparations

Calciferol injection	300,000 units/ml
Calciferol solution	3,000 units/ml
Calciferol tablets	50,000 units/1·25 mg tablet
Cholecalciferol	40,000 units/1 mg tablet
Dihydrotachysterol	0·25 mg/ml.

Pharmacology. Vitamin D is absorbed orally or by intramuscular injections, it is fat soluble and requires bile acids for absorption from the gut. The principle action is to increase the absorption of calcium from the gut and the resorption of calcium from bone, effects which are mediated through changes in protein metabolism and closely linked to the action of parathyroid hormone.

Therapeutic uses and dosages of Calciferol

Prevention of rickets	400 units per day
Treatment of rickets	3,000–4,000 units per day
Treatment of osteomalacia	5,000–50,000 units per day
Treatment of vitamin resistant rickets	up to 500,000 units per day
Hypoparathyroidism	50,000–500,000 units per day.

Dihydrotachysterol has only 25 per cent of the antirackitic activity of calciferol, but the same serum calcium raising ability, and is therefore the treatment of choice in hypoparathyroidism. The dose is 3 ml daily until the serum calcium is normal, thereafter reducing to a maintenance dose of about 1 ml daily.

Side effects. Overdosage with vitamin D will produce metastatic calcification and renal failure, early symptoms are lassitude, thirst, nausea and vomiting. Convulsions and coma are also complications of acute hypercalcaemia.

Calcium

Preparations

Oral:	Parenteral:
Calcium gluconate tablets	Calcium gluconate injection I.M. or I.V.
Effervescent calcium gluconate	Calcium chloride I.V. only
Calcium lactate tablets	Calcium lactate S.C., I.M. or I.V.

Therapeutic uses. Tetany (associated with hypoparathyroidism, rickets, chronic renal disease and coeliac disease). Hypoparathyroidism, Acute colic associated with lead poisoning, Hypocalcaemic convulsions, Asystolic cardiac arrest, Osteoporosis.

The dose is 5–20 ml of a 10 per cent solution parenterally for emergency use, or 3–15 grams orally.

Contraindications. Intravenous calcium should be given with caution to a patient on digitalis.

Side effects. Symptoms of hypercalcaemia, metastatic calcification which may progress to renal failure.

HYPOGLYCAEMIC DRUGS

Insulin preparations

Pharmacology. Insulin causes a fall in blood glucose concentration by increasing the entry of glucose into cells, and by reducing the output of glucose by the liver. In addition, insulin stimulates fat and glycogen synthesis, and decreases protein synthesis. It is not absorbed orally, being broken down by the gastric secretions.

Therapeutic uses. Insulin sensitive diabetes mellitus.

Diabetic hyperglycaemic coma.

In the insulin tolerance test to assess the integrity of the pituitary gland.

In the emergency treatment of hyperkalaemia.

Insulin has been used in the treatment of myocardial infarction, but its place is not established.

The dose in diabetes mellitis will vary from person to person, depending on the amount of endogenous insulin production, the diet and

Preparation	Animal Source	Onset	Peak	Duration
		(Hours, approx.)*		
Short acting				
Insulin injection (soluble) (UK) ⎫	Beef/pork or	½	3–6	6–8
Regular insulin (USA) ⎭	mixture		hrs	hrs
Neutral insulin injection (Actrapid)	Pork			
Insulin zinc suspension (Amorphous) (semi lente)	Beef	½	1–3	12–16
Medium acting				
Globin zinc insulin injection	Beef	1–2	6–12	18–24
Isophane insulin injection (BP) ⎫ NPH	Beef/pork or mixture	1–2	10–20	up to 28
Isophane insulin suspension (USA) ⎭				
Insulin zinc suspension (lente)	Beef/pork or mixture	2	4–5	24–28
Long acting				
Protamine zinc insulin injection (BP) ⎫ PZI	Beef/pork or mixture	4–6	8–20	24–36
Protamine zinc insulin suspension (USA) ⎭				
Insulin zinc suspension, crystalline (Ultra lente)	Beef	several hours	7–10	30+
Biphasic				
Biphasic insulin injection (Rapitard)	Mixture	½–1	4–6 / 8–24	12–24

* N.B.—An increasing dose increases the duration of action, but the figures given are representative. Individual patient variation may be over a wide range.

the amount of exercise taken. The requirements will increase in pregnancy, fever, thyrotoxicosis, infections and diabetic acidosis.

Side effects. Hypoglycaemia.

Local allergic reactions, including skin rashes, urticaria and angioneurotic oedema.

Local lipoatrophy or lipohypertrophy.

Sulphonylureas

Preparations	Relative potency	Average daily dose
Tolbutamide tablets	1 g	0·5–3 g in divided doses
Chlorpropamide	100 mg	100–500 mg daily
Tolazamide	100 mg	250–750 mg daily
Acetohexamide	200 mg	250–1,500 mg daily

Pharmacology. These preparations are absorbed by the gut, partially bound to protein and excreted via the kidney. Their main action is to release insulin from the pancreatic islet cells although in addition they may potentiate the peripheral action of insulin.

Therapeutic uses [4]. The sulphonylureas are used in the treatment of mild uncomplicated diabetes mellitus without ketonuria. They are particularly suitable for the adult type maturity onset diabetics, but should not be used to replace adequate dietary therapy. Tolbutamide given intravenously is also used as a diagnostic aid in the differential diagnosis of hypoglycaemia.

Contraindications. They are unsuitable in diabetes following total pancreatectomy, diabetes with ketosis or ketonuria, and are best avoided in children with diabetes and patients with coexistent hepatic or renal disease.

Side effects. Hypoglycaemia, particularly in the elderly and patients with hepatic or renal disease.
Leucopenia and agranulocytosis.
Skin rashes, including exfoliative dermatitis.
Cholestatic jaundice.
Gastrointestinal upsets.
Transient ataxia and muscle weakness.
Vasomotor disturbances with flushing, giddiness, tachycardia and breathlessness which may be precipitated by alcohol.
Eosinophilic pulmonary infiltrations.
Microgranulosis of the heart, liver and kidney have been described.
There may be biochemical evidence of hypothyroidism, but clinical myxoedema is rare.

Biguanides

Preparations	Average daily dose
Phenformin hydrochloride tablets	25–150 mg in divided doses
Phenformin hydrochloride SA tablets	50–150 mg
Metformin hydrochloride	1–3 g. in divided doses
Buformin hydrochloride tablets	50–300 mg in divided doses
Buformin hydrochloride SA tablets	100–300 mg

Pharmacology [5]. The exact mode of action is not established but probably the increased peripheral utilisation of both insulin and glucose is the major one.

The action of phenformin lasts 6–8 hours and that of metformin 8–12 hours, they are both excreted largely unchanged in the urine.

Therapeutic uses. As for sulphonyl ureas. In addition, the biguanides have been used as an adjuvent to insulin therapy, where smooth control has proved particularly difficult, and in the treatment of obesity in diabetics. The starting dose should always be low and gradually increased to control the blood sugar.

Contraindications. As for sulphonylureas.

Side effects

Gastrointestinal upsets, a metallic taste in the mouth, general malaise and weight loss, ketonuria without hyperglycaemia, skin rashes, lactic acidosis with phenformin.

CORTICOSTEROIDS

Pharmacology. The steroids produced by the adrenal cortex and the synthetic products can be classified into three groups on the basis of their predominant physiological effects. These are the glucocorticoids (i.e. principally affecting carbohydrate metabolism), mineralocorticoids (i.e. mainly affecting sodium and potassium metabolism), and the sex hormones which will be dealt with in a later section.

The glucocorticoids increase gluconeogenesis, inhibit peripheral utilisation of glucose and increase glycogen deposit in the liver. In addition to these effects on carbohydrate metabolism, they help to maintain normal renal function and raise the arterial blood pressure. In normal pharmacological doses they reduce the inflammatory res-

Preparations name	Equivalent oral dose	Route	Salt retaining activity
Hydrocortisone (UK) ⎫ Cortisol (USA) ⎭	20 mg	Oral/I.M./I.V.	++
Cortisone	25 mg	Oral/I.M./I.V.	++
Prednisolone	5 mg	Oral/I.M./I.V.	+
Prednisone	5 mg	Oral	+
Methyl prednisolone	4 mg	Oral/I.V./I.M.	
Paramethasone	2 mg	Oral	
Dexamethasone	0·75 mg	Oral/I.V./I.M.	
Betamethasone	0·75 mg	Oral/I.V./I.M.	
Fludrocortisone		Oral	++++
Aldosterone		I.M./I.V.	++++

ponses, decrease antibody production, and stimulate production of gastric and peptic secretion.

Mineralocorticoids

Corticosteroids with predominant mineralocorticoid activity increase the transport of sodium into cells in exchange for potassium. The principle effect of this is an increased urinary loss of potassium, with sodium retention within the body.

Therapeutic uses [6]. The corticosteroids are used therapeutically in three main categories.

1. *As substitution therapy.* In adrenocortical failure, in hypopituitarism and in congenital adrenal hyperplasia. The doses required are those which maintain normal health, electrolyte balance and arterial blood pressure. In primary adrenocortical failure, a powerful mineralocorticoid such as fludrocortisone (0·05–0·2 mg daily) is normally required in addition to cortisone (25–75 mg daily), whereas in hypopituitarism and congenital adrenal hyperplasia, cortisone alone is sufficient.

2. *In the treatment of some haematological disorders,* such as autoimmune haemolytic anaemia, idiopathic thrombocytopenic purpura, and some forms of leukaemia, especially in children.

3. *To suppress unwanted inflammatory responses* in a wide variety of disease processes. These include systemic lupus erythematosus, asthma,

dermatomyositis, polymyalgia rheumatica, cranial arteritis, poly-arteritis nodosa, selected cases of rheumatoid arthritis and the nephrotic syndrome, and occasionally in tuberculosis.

The preparation chosen in the latter two categories is one having the minimal mineralocorticoid activity. The dose may be very high for a short period (e.g. Prednisone 60–100 mg daily) in the early phase of the disease or during a relapse. But the correct dose at all times is the smallest dose necessary to produce a therapeutic response.

Side effects

Endocrine. Production of iatrogenic Cushing's syndrome.
Hyperglycaemia with accentuation or precipitation of diabetes.
Retardation of growth rate in children.
Salt and water retention with hypertension.
Potassium loss.
Mobilisation of calcium with osteoporosis.
Aseptic necrosis of the femoral head.
Suppression of the pituitary adrenal axis.

Infections. Reactivation or aggravation of tuberculosis.
Increased susceptibility to viral, bacterial, fungal and parasitic in-fections.

Eyes. Exacerbation of infections which may lead to corneal perforation.
Precipitation of glaucoma.
Cataract formation.

Skin. Atrophy with the production of striae.
Purpura.
Hypertrichosis and acne.

Gastrointestinal. There is an increased incidence of peptic ulceration and perforation.
Acute pancreatitis.
Increased incidence of toxic megacolon and perforation of ulcerative colitis.

Nervous system. Euphoria and psychosis.
Precipitation of latent epilepsy.
Raised intracranial pressure and papilloedema in children.
Pelvic girdle myopathy, especially with steroids having a F^+ ion at the 9a position.

Contraindications. The contraindications are all relative, depending on the severity of the disease for which they are to be used. However, they should rarely be used when the following conditions are present:

Peptic ulcer	Diabetes
Osteoporosis	Active or possibly active
Psychosis	tuberculosis
Congestive cardiac failure	Acute systemic viral or bacterial
	infections

Corticotrophin

Preparations

Short acting:

Corticotrophin injection (UK) – I.V. or I.M. preparation.

Corticotropin injection (USA) – I.M. preparation.

Long acting

Corticotrophin gelatin injection (UK).

Repository Corticotropin injection (USA).

Corticotrophin zinc hydroxide injection (UK).

Sterile Corticotropin zinc hydroxide suspension (USA).

Corticotrophin-carboxymethyl cellulose complex (ACTH/CMC).

Synthetic

Tetracosactrin (B^{1-24} corticotrophin).

Tetracosactrin depot.

Pharmacology. Corticotrophin stimulates the production and release of adrenal steroids. It also has some melanocyte stimulating action by virtue of the structural similarity to MSH, and suppresses corticotrophin releasing factor both by the production of high levels of corticosteroids and by direct action on the hypothalamus.

Therapeutic use. Stimulation of the adrenals following long-term corticosteroid therapy.

Asthma in children during the growing period

Bell's palsy

Multiple sclerosis.

Corticotrophin is always given parenterally. A maximal response is obtained with 40 I.U. twice daily, but the dose should always be the minimal needed to control the disease. It is better to give a larger dose less frequently (e.g. twice weekly) than a small dose daily.

Diagnostic uses [7]. Corticotrophin is used to assess the function of the adrenal cortex by measuring either the plasma cortisol or the urinary 17-hydroxycorticoids response following stimulation with corticotrophin. More recently the synthetic preparations have been used with more consistent results.

Contraindications and side effects. As for corticosteroids with the addition of pigmentation, which may occur during treatment with both natural and synthetic corticotrophin, and the occasional allergic response.

ANABOLIC STEROIDS

Preparations	Dose (mg/kg)	Route
Nandrolone phenylpropionate	0·75–1·0/week	I.M.
Nandrolone decanoate	1·0 –1·5/4 weeks	I.M.
Methenolone oenanthate	1·0 –2·0/10 days	I.M.
Norethandrolone	0·5 –1·0/day	Oral
Methandienone	0·2 –0·3/day	Oral
Methendone acetate	0·4 –0·6/day	Oral
Oxymetholone	0·25–0·5/day	Oral
Stanozolol	0·1 –0·15/day	Oral
Ethyloestrenol	0·05–0·1/day	Oral

Pharmacology. These compounds result from attempts to alter the chemical structure of the androgens, so as to reduce the androgenic effects and retain their protein anabolic function. At the present time all these drugs retain some virilising properties. Apart from causing nitrogen retention they also increase the retention of calcium sodium, potassium, chloride and phosphate ions and increase bone growth and maturation.

Therapeutic uses. There is no universal agreement regarding the indications for the anabolic steroids. Generally they are less effective in men than in women, they are rarely useful in acute catabolic diseases, and there is no indication for their use as a 'tonic'. They may contribute to nitrogen retention and protein anabolism in chronic debilitating diseases post-menopausal and senile osteoporosis and chronic renal failure [8]. They should be used with care in growth retardation, as epiphyseal closure may exceed increase in bone growth. Their place in the treatment of corticosteroid osteoporosis, burns and acute renal failure is not established.

Side effects

Virilising. This may occur in females with any preparation, and some patients appear to be excessively sensitive to this effect.

Hepatic. As with the androgens, those which have 17α alkyl substitution (the orally active preparations) cause liver impairment and may produce a reversible cholestatic jaundice.

Others. The oral preparations may also cause a rise in serum cholesterol and lipids, especially in conjunction with corticosteroids or in non-insulin requiring diabetics. Contraindications are the same as for androgens.

PROGESTOGENS

Preparations	Dose to produce a secretory endometrium
Progesterone injection (UK) ⎫ Progesterone suspension (USA) ⎭	50–100 mg I.M. daily for five days
Progesterone derivatives	
Dydrogesterone tablets (UK) ⎫ Didrogesterone tablets (USA) ⎭	10 mg daily orally for 10–15 days
Hydroprogesterone Caproate	250 mg I.M.
Chlormanidone acetate	2 mg orally for 2 days
Medroxyprogesterone acetate	10 mg daily for 10 days orally. 50 mg I.M. once
19 *Nortestosterone derivatives*	
Norethisterone (UK) ⎫ Norethindrome (USA) ⎭	10–30 mg daily orally for 10 days
Norethynodrel tablets	10–30 mg daily orally for 10 days
Dimethesterone tablets	15–40 mg daily orally for 10 days
Ethynodial diacetate	1–2 mg daily orally for 10 days

Pharmacology. The progestogens produce the secretory changes in the endometrium, maturation of breast prior to lactation, and progesterone is responsible for the rise in basal temperature following ovulation, and the maintenance of normal pregnancy.

Therapeutic uses. The treatment of functional uterine bleeding.
   Premenstrual tension.
   Contraception.

Endometriosis.

In the diagnosis of amenorrhoea.

Progestogens have also been used in the treatment of habitual and threatened abortion, but their value is doubtful.

Side effects. All progestogens may cause nausea, vomiting and weight gain. The nortestosterone derivatives are variably androgenic, and consequently can cause hirsutism, acne and deepening of the voice. If given during pregnancy, virilisation of the foetus can occur. The progestogens with an alkyl group in the 17α position (Norethisterone, Norethynodrel) may cause cholestatic jaundice, and should be avoided in patients with liver disease.

OESTROGENS

Pharmacology. Oestrogens stimulate the development and maintain the secondary sexual characteristics including stromal and duct growth in the breast. They are responsible for the proliferation of the endometrium, and for the cyclic changes of the cervix and vagina. The pubertal growth spurt and epiphyseal closure is also an oestrogenic effect. There are a number of other general metabolic effects involving protein, fat, glucose and phosphate metabolism, and salt and water retention. Oestrogens increase the proteins which bind corticosteroids and thyroxine, which may give rise to difficulty in interpreting plasma levels of cortisol and protein bound iodine. There are also effects on the blood clotting factors.

Therapeutic uses. Replacement therapy in primary or secondary ovarian failure.

Suppression of lactation.

Suppression of ovulation in dysmenorrhoea.

With progestogens as a contraceptive.

With progestogens in the treatment of endometriosis.

Metropathic uterine bleeding.

Delayed puberty.

To encourage epiphyseal closure when there is excessive growth in girls.

Control of menopausal symptoms.

Treatment of carcinoma of the breast and prostate.

The dose will depend on the condition and will also vary with the patient. Examples of ethinyl oestradiol are 0·01–0·05 mg daily for menopausal symptoms; 0·05–0·25 mg daily in replacement therapy and the treatment of primary amenorrhoea; to control metropathic

Preparations	Usual dose	Route
Ethinyl oestradiol (UK) Ethinyl Estradiol (USA)	0·05–0·2 mg daily	Oral
Oestradiol (UK) Estradiol (USA)	0·25–10 mg daily 50–300 mg 4–6 monthly	Oral By implantation
Oestradiol benzoate (UK) Estradiol benzoate (USA)	1–5 mg 1–3 times weekly	I.M.
Oestradiol cypionate (UK) Estradiol cypionate (USA)	1–5 mg every 3–4 weeks	I.M.
Oestradiol Dipropionate (UK) Estradiol Dipropionate (USA)	1–5 mg weekly	I.M.
Oestradiol Valerate (UK) Estradiol Valerate (USA)	5–20 mg every 2–4 weeks	I.M.
Piperazine Oestrone Sulphate (UK) Piperazine Estrone Sulphate (USA)	0·75–4·5 mg daily	Oral
Oestrogenic substances, conjugated	0·125–2·5 mg daily 20 mg	Oral I.V.
Non-steroidal Oestrogens		
Stilboestrol (UK) Diethyl stilboestrol (USA)	0·5–10 mg daily	Oral or I.M.
Stilboestrol Diphosphate (UK) Diethyl stilboestrol Diphosphate (USA)	250 mg–1 g. (Treatment of prostate carcinoma)	I.V.
Dienoestrol (UK) Dienestrol (USA)	0·1–5 mg daily	Oral
Chlorotrianisene	12–48 mg daily	Oral
Methallenoestril (UK) Methallenestril (USA)	3–9 mg daily	Oral

bleeding 0·5–2 mg daily should be given until the bleeding stops, or 20 mg of conjugated oestrogens may be given intravenously in an emergency; 0·1 mg three times daily is given to terminate lactation. The highest doses are given in the treatment of carcinoma of the prostate, when doses up to 10 mg or more are given daily.

Side effects. Nausea, headache, breast tenderness and weight gain due to sodium and water retention are frequent, usually transient, effects. More serious is the occurrence of thromboembolic phenomena. Oestrogens should be avoided in patients particularly liable to thromboembolism, in renal disease congestive cardiac failure and neoplasms of the female genital tract.

Androgens

Preparations	Dose/Route and frequency
Testosterone implants (UK) ⎱ Testosterone pellets (USA) ⎰	200–1000 mg by subcutaneous implantation every 4–8 months
Testosterone propionate	5–25 mg intramuscularly one to two times each week
Testosterone phenylpropionate	10–100 mg weekly intramuscularly
Testosterone oenanthate (UK) ⎱ Testosterone enanthate (USA) ⎰	100–200 mg intramuscularly every 2–4 weeks
Testosterone cypionate	10–100 mg intramuscularly every 1–2 weeks
Methyl testosterone tablets	25–50 mg sublingually daily
Fluoxymesterone	5–20 mg sublingually daily

Pharmacology. Testosterone and other androgenic steroids are responsible for the normal development of secondary sexual characteristics in the male. They also produce marked nitrogen retention and protein anabolism, which results in the growth spurt at puberty. They also cause maturation of bones, with fusion of the epiphyses.

Therapeutic uses. The only clear cut indication of the use of androgens is in the treatment of primary or secondary male hypogonadism. Either a long acting preparation such as testosterone oenanthate or testosterone implants are the most suitable preparations. While it is possible to get good sexual development there is rarely any improvement in spermatogenesis.

Androgens have also been used in the treatment of carcinoma of the breast in females, aplastic anaemia, osteoporosis and growth disorders, but the value and indications are not well established.

Side effects and contraindications. A reversible cholestatic type of jaundice may occur with the androgens which are substituted in the 17α position (methyl testosterone and Fluoxymesterone). This is a dose related not a sensitivity effect.

Other side effects include the suppression of spermatogenesis, sodium and water retention, hypercalcaemia and virilisation if administered to females.

Androgens are absolutely contraindicated in pregnancy and carcinoma of the prostate. They should be used with special care in children, and when there is hepatic or renal disease.

References

1. Gemzell, C. A., Roos, P., and Loeffler, E. E., *J. Reprod. Fertil* (1966), **12**, 49–64. The clinical use of pituitary gonadotrophins in women.

2. Roy, S., Greenblatt, R. B., Mahesh, V. B., and Jungck, E. C., *Fertil and Steril* (1963), **14**, 575. Clomiphene citrate: Further observations on its mode of action.

3. Astwood, E. P., *Thyrotoxicosis*. Proceedings of symposium Edinburgh (1969), Editor Irvine, W. J., Livingstone.

4. Madsen, J., *Acta med. Scand.* (1967), Suppl. 476, 108. The intrahepatic and extrapancreatic actions of sulphonylureas: A review.

5. Butterfield, W. J. H., *Ann. N.Y. Acad. Sci.* (1968), **148**, 724.

6. Picton, T., *Guide to Steroid Therapy* (1968), London, Lloyd-Luke.

7. Mattingly, D., *Proceedings of the Fourth Symposium on advanced medicine*, (1968), (ed. O. Wrong), London, Pitman.

8. Wynn, V., *Anabolic steroids and protein metabolism* (1967). In modern trends in endocrinology, (ed. Gardner-Hill), London, Butterworths.

This Chapter was written by Dr. M. N. Maisey (Dept of Endocrinology, Guy's Hospital) and edited by Prof. J. R. Trounce.

Category 14

Miscellaneous Drugs

THE CHELATING AGENTS

Desferrioxamine

Pharmacological action. This drug is an iron-free compound obtained from ferrioxamine, a metabolite of *Streptomyces pilosus*. It is an iron-complexing agent capable of eliminating iron from the body. It does not remove iron from haemoglobin or iron-containing enzymes. The iron complex formed with such substances as ferritin, haemosiderin and transferrin is rapidly excreted by the kidneys. The serum iron concentration quickly decreases. The drug has almost exclusive affinity for iron.

Therapeutic use [1]. The drug is of value in secondary haemochromatosis, e.g. in aplastic anaemia, transfusion haemosiderosis, sickle cell anaemia and severe chronic acquired haemolytic anaemia. The dose is 1 g daily in one or two intramuscular injections; for maintenance purposes 500 mg is given daily.

Desferrioxamine is of great value in the treatment of children who have taken an overdose of iron tablets. After gastric lavage with bicarbonate solution desferrioxamine should be instilled into the stomach, suggested doses being 3–7 g. in 50–200 ml of water or saline. This will prevent absorption of any iron still present in the gastrointestinal tract. At the same time an intravenous drip should be set up and desferrioxamine infused in a maximum dose of 15 mg/kg of bodyweight/hour to a total of 80 mg/kg bodyweight. Desferrioxamine is rapidly absorbed from muscle and it may be wise to give 2 g. I.M. before starting the time-consuming gastric lavage and intravenous infusion.

Side effects. Pain occurs at the site of intramuscular injection. The volume of urine may be temporarily decreased. The serum calcium is sometimes decreased.

Dimercaprol (British Anti-Lewisite)

Pharmacological action. The drug rapidly enters the circulation within five minutes after intramuscular injection; it is rapidly distributed and eliminated within a few hours. The greater part of the drug is quickly metabolised and excreted in the urine. The dithiol forms relatively stable chelated complexes with arsenic, mercury, gold, and certain other metals. It is also highly effective locally.

Therapeutic use. The drug has been shown to be of value in arsenical intoxication, mercuric chloride poisoning and in toxic reactions due to gold.

In hepatolenticular degeneration it increases the already high copper output in the urine, causing some improvement in the disease.

The drug is given as a 5 per cent solution of dimercaprol in arachis oil with benzylbenzoate as solubiliser. Administration is by intramuscular injection 8–16 ml in divided doses on the first day; 4–8 ml in divided doses on the second and third days; and 2–4 ml in divided doses on subsequent days.

Side effects. Reactions are of minor importance, reversible, and of short duration; they usually occur with doses exceeding 3 mg per kg of bodyweight. They may be prevented by giving an antihistaminic drug or ephedrine beforehand. Paraesthesiae, pains or burning of the mouth, eyes, feet, sweating, lacrimation, salivation, vomiting, weakness, rise in systolic and diastolic blood pressure; these features last thirty to sixty minutes.

Care is required in patients with impaired liver function. Renal damage may be produced due to excretion of the drug with chelated metal. The intramuscular injection may cause severe local necrosis. Intravenous injection may cause cardiac collapse.

Sodium calcium edetate

Pharmacological action. The drug forms strong un-ionised complexes with cations. The calcium compound is used to avoid producing low-calcium tetany.

Therapeutic use [2, 3]. The drug is effective in acute and chronic lead poisoning; it produces a marked increase in the urinary excretion of lead. In hepatolenticular degeneration it has been given with dimercaprol to increase the copper output in the urine. In digitalis intoxication and certain other arrhythmias sodium edetate has been used to bind calcium ions.

It is given by intravenous infusion, a maximum of 40 mg per kg bodyweight being given daily usually in two doses given over a period of one hour. A course of treatment usually lasts three days.

Pencillamine

Pharmacological action. This chelating agent consists of a portion of the penicillin molecule, which is an analogue of the aminoacid cysteine. In copper, lead and iron poisoning it appears to increase the excretion of these metals.

Therapeutic use. The drug is effective in hepatolenticular degeneration in promoting cupruresis. It has been used in copper, lead and iron poisoning.

Penicillamine hydrochloride is given in capsule form, 0·9–1·5 g. daily, in divided doses, before meals.

Side effects. It may produce morbilliform skin rashes, and renal damage has been reported. Agranulocytosis may occur.

ANALEPTICS

This group of drugs are central stimulants with a marked effect on the medulla. They were formerly used to reverse the effect of medullary depressive drugs, in particular the barbiturates, but it is now realised that their use is of doubtful value in treating barbiturate overdosage. They are also occasionally used in increasing ventilation in those with respiratory failure.

The main members of the group are:

	Dose	Uses
Picrotoxin	In barbiturate poisoning 6·0 mg at a rate of 1 mg/minute I.V.	Powerful central stimulant can produce convulsions, very short-acting.
Leptazol	In barbiturate poisoning up to 1·0 ml of a 10 per cent solution I.V.	Powerful central stimulant can produce convulsions, very short-acting.
Nikethamide	2–8 ml of 25 per cent solution I.V.	Less powerful central effect. Also sensitises carotid body. Very short-acting.
Amiphenazole	100–200 mg t.d.s., oral or 100 mg I.M.	Milder and longer-acting.
Bemegride	In barbiturate poisoning 50 mg I.V. repeated if necessary at intervals of 10 minutes to a total of 1·0 g.	Longer-acting.

APPETITE SUPPRESSORS

Phenmetrazine

Diethylpropion

Pharmacological action and therapeutic uses. These drugs are powerful suppressors of appetite with minimal adrenergic effect. They are used in the treatment of obesity. The dose is

Phenmetrazine   12·5–25 mg b.d.

Diethylpropion   25 mg t.d.s.

Contraindications and side effects. Dependence can occur with both these drugs. They should not be used in the early part of pregnancy, for there is some circumstantial evidence [4] that one of them (phenmetrazine) may affect the foetus.

Fenfluramine

Pharmacology and therapeutic use. Fenfluramine depresses appetite without apparently any stimulating effect on the central nervous system. In fact it sometimes has a mild sedative action. It is fairly long-acting and the recommended dose in obesity is 1 tablet (20 mg) two hours before the evening meal and 1 tablet mid-morning, but up to six tablets can be given daily. The main side effect is diarrhoea, with occasional nausea. Overdosage however, can produce agitation, confusion, convulsions and death.

THE ANTIHISTAMINES

The antihistamines are a large group of drugs, which in general are very similar in their actions, although they differ as to which particular action predominates.

Pharmacological action. The antihistamines are well absorbed from the gut and largely metabolised in the liver.

Their main pharmacological actions are:

1. They are competitive blockers of all the actions of histamine except they do not prevent histamine induced gastric secretion.

2. They are usually CNS depressors, producing some drowsiness and also are antiemetics.

3. They have some mild peripheral anticholinergic action.

4. They have a weak effect on the heart, similar to that of quinidine.

Therapeutic uses. Antihistamines are used in various allergic conditions, including urticaria and hay fever. They are rarely effective in bronchial asthma. Their effect on the CNS is used to prevent vomiting and they also may reduce the symptoms of Parkinson's disease.

Individual preparations

(a) Useful as antihistamines:

Promethazine: long-acting 25–50 mg at night often sufficient. Sedation marked.

Diphenhydramine: 25–50 mg four times daily. Sedation marked.

Mepyramine: 100–200 mg three times daily.

Chlorpheniramine: 4 mg three times daily or 10 mg I.M. Good antihistamine effect, some sedation.

Phenindamine: 25–50 mg three times daily. Little if any sedation.

(b) Useful as antiemetics:

Dimenhydrinate: 50 mg four times daily. Sedation marked.

Cyclizine: 50 mg three times daily. Mild sedation.

Meclozine: 50 mg daily. Mild sedation.

Promethazine chlorotheophyllinate: 25 mg three times daily. Quite marked sedation.

Vomiting in pregnancy. All drugs should be avoided in early pregnancy, if possible. However, it is fair to say that the antiemetics listed above have not been shown to produce foetal abnormalities.

Contraindications and side effects. Troublesome sedation is the commonest side effect. The anticholinergic action of these drugs may produce dry mouth and gastrointestinal upsets. Rarely they produce bone marrow depression. It is interesting that both systemic and local use can produce sensitisation rashes.

Disodium cromoglycate

Pharmacology. Disodium cromoglycate is thought to relieve bronchospasm in asthma by inhibiting the release of bronchoconstrictor substances which follows an antigen-antibody union. It is not an antispasmodic. It is poorly absorbed from the gut and is given by inhalation.

Therapeutic use. Disodium cromoglycate is used to prevent attacks of asthma. It is given by inhalation and there are two formulations: either 20 mg disodium cromoglycate per Spincap capsule or 20 mg of disodium cromoglycate and 0·1 mg of isoprenaline per Spincap capsule. Initial treatment is one capsule night and morning and at 4–6-hourly intervals – this can be reduced when a satisfactory response is obtained. Disodium cromoglycate can be given concurrently with steroid or antispasmodics and may enable the dose of steroids to be reduced. If disodium cromoglycate is suddenly withdrawn in those whose steroid dose has been reduced the dose of sterioids must be returned to their previous level or a severe relapse of asthma can occur.

Metoclopramide

Pharmacological action. Metoclopramide is an antiemetic but not an antihistamine. Its mode of action is not clear, but it decreases gastric emptying time, probably by stimulation of autonomic ganglia, and relaxes the duodenum.

Therapeutic use. Metoclopramide has been used in many types of vomiting and success has been claimed, although most of these studies are not very satisfactory. The oral dose is 10 mg and can be given three times daily. It can also be given intramuscularly in doses of 10 mg.

Contraindications and side effects. Metoclopramide can produce drowsiness with large doses. Dystonia has been reported and it should not be combined therefore with the phenothiazines. It should not be given in the first three months of pregnancy.

ANTACIDS

Antacids are used to relieve the pain of peptic ulcers. There is no evidence that they alter the rate of healing of an ulcer. They act by raising the pH of the gastric contents and thereby reducing the irritant effect of the gastric acid on the ulcer and decreasing the activity of pepsin. This is achieved if the pH of the gastric content is raised to around 4·0. The most widely used antacids are:

Sodium bicarbonate

Sodium bicarbonate is a rapidly acting antacid, but passes quickly through the stomach so its action is transient. It is absorbed and can thus produce alkalosis, although this does not occur with usual doses if renal function is normal. It is usually given in a dose of 1·0 g. mixed with a little water.

Magnesium oxide

This salt is rather longer acting than sodium bicarbonate. There is no danger of alkalosis but all magnesium salts cause diarrhoea due to the poor absorption of the magnesium ion. The dose of magnesium oxide is 0·3–0·6 g.

Magnesium trisilicate
A white powder given orally in a dose of 1·0 g. mixed with milk or water. Much slower in action and longer activity than the previous magnesium salts. In order to spread the action of magnesium salts they are often combined in a single tablet.

Calcium carbonate
This is an efficient antacid in doses of 1–2 g. It is important to remember that calcium carbonate combined with excessive milk intake can cause hypercalcaemia in some individuals leading to thirst, polyurea and renal damage.

Aluminium hydroxide
Aluminium hydroxide is a useful antacid and can be given either as a gel or in tablet form. It is said to have some inhibiting effect on pepsin.

Carbenoxolone
Pharmacology and therapeutic use. Carbenoxolone is a turpene. There is good evidence that it increases the rate of healing of gastric ulcers in ambulant patients. Its usefulness in duodenal ulcers is not as yet proven. Its mode of action is not known but it provides increased secretion of mucous by the stomach and this may protect the ulcer. The usual dose is 50–100 mg t.d.s. It can cause sodium and water retention and should not be used in those in or near cardiac failure, and care should be taken in the elderly. It can also rarely cause potassium depletion and muscle weakness. Carbenoxolene should not be used for more than two months.

PURGATIVES

Liquid paraffin. Acts by its lubricating action. It is useful particularly in the elderly and in painful conditions of the lower bowel. The dose is 15 ml twice daily or 5·0 ml, hourly for a few hours. Prolonged administration can cause vitamin A and D deficiency and inhalation by the very young or very ill can cause a paraffinoma in the lung.

Bulk purges. These act by increasing the bowel contents. There are a number of preparations available containing agar (dose: 4–8 g.) or methylcellulese (dose: 1–1·5 g.).

Saline purges. Magnesium sulphate is widely used in a dose of 8·0 g. in 150 ml of water before breakfast.

IRRITANT PURGES

Phenolphthalein
Pharmacology. Phenolphthalein is absorbed from the intestine and stimulates the colon. It is re-excreted via the bile and so a certain amount of recirculation occurs.

Therapeutic uses and side effects. Phenolphthalein in a dose of 120 mg at bedtime produces a purge the next morning. It is relatively free of side effects but can produce rashes.

Anthracene purges
Pharmacology. This group of purges contains a number of substances including emodin, which stimulates the colon.

Therapeutic uses
Senna – best given as the Senokot containing the purified active principles. The adult dose is 2–4 tablets or 1–2 teaspoonfuls of granules.
Cascara – Tablets of cascara (BP) 125–250 mg.

OTHER PURGATIVES

Bisacodyl
This purgative stimulates the colon when it comes into contact with the bowel wall. The dose is 5–10 mg.

Dioctyl-sodium sulphosuccinate
This substance is a wetting agent and softens the bowel contents. It is useful in faecal impaction in doses of 40–60 mg three times daily.

References
1. Williams, R., *Recent advances in medicine* (1968), Churchill, London.
2. Sapeika, N., *Actions and uses of drugs* (1966), Balkema, Capetown.
3. Browning, E., *Toxicity of industrial metals* (1969), 2nd ed., Butterworth, London.
4. Powell, P. D., and Johnstone, J. M., *Brit. med. J.* (1962), **ii**, 1327.

This chapter was written by Prof. J. R. Trounce.

Category 15

Vitamins

Vitamin A (Retinol, *USA*)
Pharmacological action. Vitamin A is required for the formation of visual purple which is essential for the eye to see in dim light. Vitamin A also directly affects the metabolism of all epithelial tissues; it appears to be necessary for the normal formation of mucopolysaccharides.

Therapeutic use [1]. Vitamin A is used for the treatment of zerophthalmia and of night blindness when this is due to dietary failure. It should also be given to malnourished people who show evidence of follicular keratosis.

Cod liver and shark liver oils are good natural concentrated sources of the vitamin. The prophylactic dose for children is 3,000 I.U. and for adults 5,000 I.U. daily. A therapeutic dose totalling 250,000 I.U. of retinol given in capsules over a period of one week usually achieves maximum therapeutic benefit.

Side effects. High doses taken by early Arctic explorers caused drowsiness, headache with increased cerebrospinal fluid pressure, vomiting and extensive peeling of the skin. Sporadic cases in children in recent years have generally been due to over-enthusiastic administration of fish liver oils. Rapid recovery follows withdrawal of the vitamin.

Vitamin D (Cholecalciferol, *USA*)
Pharmacological action. The vitamin probably has a direct action on bone; it is necessary for formation of normal bone and for the calcification of rachitic bone. The mechanism of its action on bone is uncertain. In addition it promotes the absorption of calcium and phosphate from the gut, thus ensuring a sufficient supply of the minerals to the growing points of bones.

Therapeutic use. For prophylactic use cod liver oil is the best natural source. Not more than 10 ml should be taken daily. The therapeutic dose is 4,000 to 50,000 units daily; the vitamin is used in the treatment and prevention of rickets and osteomalacia. It is also useful in correcting low levels of serum calcium such as occur in the malabsorption syndrome and in hypoparathyroidism.

Side effects. As this vitamin is fat soluble it is not rapidly metabolised or excreted. If taken in excessive amounts it may accumulate in the body and produce toxic effects. The earliest toxic symptom in children is usually sudden loss of appetite. Nausea and vomiting are frequently associated. Thirst and polyuria soon follow. There may be severe constipation, alternating with bouts of diarrhoea. Headache and other pains are frequent. The child may become thin, wan, irritable, depressed and gradually fall into a stuporose condition which may suggest meningitis. In fatal cases metastatic calcification has been found at autopsy in the arteries, renal tubules, heart, lungs and elsewhere. The serum calcium may be elevated to 12 mg/100 ml or more, but it may remain normal.

Vitamin K (Menaphthon, *USA*)

Pharmacological action. The vitamin is necessary for the normal formation of prothrombin in the liver; the manner in which vitamin K participates in this process is not understood.

Therapeutic use. The vitamin is given to neonates in order to prevent bleeding in a newborn infant who has suffered from trauma at birth, or who shows signs of bleeding. In underdeveloped countries where haemorrhagic disease of the newborn is an important problem there is a strong case for prophylactic use of vitamin K_1 as a routine. The dose for a baby is 1 mg of vitamin K_1 (phytomenadione) intramuscularly, repeated in eight hours if necessary.

In cases of biliary obstruction and fistula, and in malabsorption, if surgery is contemplated, vitamin K_1 is essential pre-operatively for three days in a dose of 10 to 20 mg daily intramuscularly. When there is severe liver damage little or no improvement in the prothrombin level in the blood can be expected unless a blood transfusion is given.

In anticoagulant therapy with the phenindione group of drugs the 'prothrombin time' may increase to the point when bleeding results. In severe cases 20 mg of phytomenadione can be injected intravenously and repeated in four hours if the 'prothrombin time' has not returned to a safe level. In less severe cases the drug can be given by mouth (10–20 mg every eight hours).

Vitamin C (ascorbic acid)

Pharmacological action. Ascorbic acid maintains a healthy state of the capillary walls and the intercellular substance. It is a hydrogen transport agent in oxidation–reduction systems.

Therapeutic use. Ascorbic acid has specific effects in the treatment of scurvy. The aim should be to saturate the body with as little delay as possible;

250 mg by mouth four times daily should achieve this within a week.
Side effects. Synthetic ascorbic acid is harmless even in large doses.

Vitamin B₁ (thiamine)

Pharmacological action. The pyrophosphate of thiamine is the coenzyme of carboxylase, the enzyme concerned with the decarboxylation and oxidation of pyruvic acid. The normal function of nerve cells and the kidney is dependent on this vitamin.

Therapeutic use. Thiamine is life-saving in the treatment of cardio-vascular and infantile beriberi, and Wernicke's encephalopathy. It may be given, though without expectation of dramatic results, in cases of nutritional neuropathy. 25–100 mg daily for several weeks is required in the treatment of thiamine deficiency. Intramuscular injection may be efficacious where oral therapy fails.

Riboflavine (Vitamin B₂)

Pharmacological action. Riboflavine is present in the prosthetic groups of the flavo-proteins, essential for cellular oxidation.

Therapeutic use. There are no incontrovertible indications for the use of synthetic riboflavine; however there is probably an indication for its use in cases of malabsorption syndrome with angular stomatitis. The vitamin may be given orally or parenterally in doses of 5 mg three times daily.

Side effects. No side effects of treatment with riboflavine have been described.

Nicotinic acid (niacin)

Pharmacological action. Nicotinic acid amide is required for the action of NADH and NADPH (prosthetic groups in certain tissue oxidising enzymes).

Therapeutic use. Nicotinic acid and nicotinamide have specific and dramatic effects in pellagra and in secondary deficiency in malabsorption syndromes. The therapeutic dose is 50–250 mg daily (orally or by injection). Large doses produce a generalised and transient vasodilatation.

References

1. Davidson, S., and Passmore, R., *Human Nutrition and Dietetics* (1969), Livingstone, London.

This chapter was written by Dr P. I. Folb (Dept of Clinical Pharmacology, Guy's Hospital Medical School) and edited by Prof. J. R. Trounce.

Category 16

Vaccines and Sera

Smallpox vaccine

Pharmacological action. The vaccine is prepared from vaccinia (cowpox) virus. It is applied to the scarified skin, or by pressure inoculation of the skin, and it produces the local and general reactions of cowpox, and confers immunity for many years against smallpox.

Therapeutic use [1]. Ideally, vaccination might be carried out at four to six months of age depending on the infant immunisation programme and should be repeated on entering school, and at 5 to 10 year intervals thereafter, or at any time that exposure to smallpox is suspected. International travel requirements demand a three-year revaccination programme.

Three types of reaction to vaccination are recognised, depending on host susceptibility: (a) primary reaction, or 'take'; (b) an accelerated reaction, seen in partially immune individuals; (c) an immune reaction.

Failure to develop a reaction is not indicative of immunity and calls for revaccination with a fresh batch of vaccine.

Side effects and contraindications. 1. Generalised vaccinia. (It is not possible to know before vaccination which subjects will develop generalised vaccinia.)

2. Eczema vaccinatum. Vaccination is contraindicated in infants and others with eczema, and other forms of dermatitis; neither should these people be exposed to others who have recently been vaccinated.

3. Vaccinia gangrenosa (gangrenous vaccinia). This is an exceedingly rare complication of vaccination which is often fatal. It occurs in children with impaired mechanisms of antibody formation.

4. Congenital vaccinia may complicate vaccination during pregnancy and is possibly associated with an increased incidence of abortions. Vaccination during pregnancy is therefore contraindicated. The hazard is greater during the first and second trimester of pregnancy. (No teratogenic effect of vaccinia virus on the foetus has been demonstrated.)

5. Post-vaccinial encephalitis. The incidence of this complication in one study was 1:4,500. This incidence can be reduced by passive immunisation with antivaccinial gamma globulin at the time of primary vaccination.

Rabies vaccine

Pharmacological action. Vaccination with live, attenuated or inactivated rabies vaccine elicits antibody production in 10–14 days. This implies that vaccine therapy would be effective only where the incubation period exceeds that time. However, it is possible that antibody production is not the only mechanism of immunity and that the altered rabies virus serves to block receptor sites.

Therapeutic use [2, 3]. A course of 14 daily inoculations is usually given to an individual exposed to rabies.

Side effects and contraindications. The chief hazards of rabies vaccine are hypersensitivity reactions with severe local erythema, accompanied by fever and arthralgia in about 5 per cent of cases, and peripheral neuritis or allergic encephalomyelitis, caused by the rabbit brain tissue in which the virus is prepared, in 1 of 600 to 1 of 10,000 vaccinated individuals according to different reports. The neurological disability varies from transient neurological disturbance to permanent paralysis.

Poliomyelitis vaccine

Pharmacological action. The vaccine is prepared from strains of poliomyelitis virus. Two kinds are used; the living attenuated virus for oral administration (Sabin) and the killed vaccine (Salk). The living oral vaccine mimics the natural infection and confers the same quality of immunity; it produces local resistance to reinfection of the gut, probably a function of IgA antibodies. Circulating antibodies are also produced which limit the spread of the virus to the central nervous system. Killed virus vaccine produces high levels of circulating antibodies, initially IgM and later IgG. This probably blocks the spread of virus from the gut to the central nervous system.

Therapeutic use [4]. The three classified groups of poliomyelitis virus are given together orally as a trivalent virus, and three doses are given at intervals of about four to six weeks. Children are vaccinated at about six months of age, depending on the programme adopted. Killed vaccine is relatively little used at present.

Side effects and contraindications. Attenuated living vaccine is remarkably safe in practice. Occasionally poliomyelitis or neurovirulence of the attenuated virus have been reported.

Measles vaccine

Pharmacological action. Either killed or live attenuated measles virus is used. The antibody response after immunisation follows the same pattern as in natural measles, but the titres are slightly lower and there is a decline in antibody over a period of five or six years. Sero-conversion rates of 90–100 per cent have been obtained by vaccination of susceptible children.

Therapeutic use [4]. The vaccine is used for prophylaxis. It is given in certain programmes by intramuscular injection as inactivated vaccine, followed in four to six weeks by a single dose of live attenuated measles vaccine given by intramuscular or subcutaneous injection.

Side effects and contraindications. Few severe reactions are now encountered with the live attenuated vaccine. A mild illness with fever, rash, malaise and upper respiratory discomfort occurs in approximately 5–10 per cent of vaccinations. Occasionally there may be a very high fever.

BCG vaccine (tuberculosis vaccine)

Pharmacological action. BCG is an attenuated live vaccine derived from a virulent strain of Mycobacterium tuberculosis var bovis; the assumption is that the artificial infection will enhance resistance to subsequent infection by pathogenic mycobacterial organisms, viz. Myco. tuberculosis, Myco. leprae and Myco. ulcerans. The reason for this protection is probably due to the wide range of common antigens shared by many species of mycobacterium.

Therapeutic use [5]. In subjects not previously infected with tubercle bacilli or other mycobacteria, BCG is capable of conferring 80 per cent protection against subsequent tuberculous infection in all forms of the disease, and this protection lasts for more than 10 years. Ideally the first vaccination is given very early in life, again according to the programme adopted.

BCG vaccine has been shown to offer significant protection against the early indeterminate and tuberculoid forms of leprosy and to maintain its effect over a period of at least 44 months. There is no evidence yet that BCG vaccination protects against the lepromatous type of leprosy.

Protection against Buruli ulcer is given by BCG.

Side effects and contraindications. Modern preparations are safe and free of side effects.

Rubella vaccine

Pharmacological action. Live, attenuated rubella virus is administered; a non-transmissible and inapparent infection is produced with satisfactory antibody conversion. There is a very high rate (96–100 per cent) of seroconversion, but antibody titres are however 4-fold to 16-fold lower than those following natural infection.

Therapeutic use [4]. Administration is by vaccination. The importance of the rubella vaccine is in the prevention of infection of the foetus following maternal infection in early pregnancy. Details of the most suitable time for immunisation have still to be decided, but it might be suggested that ideally all young females should receive it before they reach reproductive age.

Side effects. Mild upper respiratory symptoms may occur following vaccination. Joint involvement with certain features in common with natural rubella has been noted; adult females are not frequently affected. It is not known whether or not the attenuated virus causes foetal damage.

Influenza vaccine

Pharmacological action. This is an aqueous suspension of inactivated but antigenic influenza virus. As a rule, the most recent strains of virus to cause epidemics and pandemics are included in the vaccine. Active immunisation is produced; protection develops in two to three weeks but is short-lived.

Therapeutic use [6]. The vaccine is administered prophylactically, as a single dose of 1 ml by deep subcutaneous injection, and aerosols are also being developed. It may be given during an epidemic, particularly to medical and nursing staff. In addition, it is given to patients at special risk, e.g. patients with chronic cardiac and pulmonary insufficiency. Vaccination must be yearly to maintain antibody levels. The limitation of the value of the vaccine is due to the multiple sero-types of the influenza viruses, and when a new serotype appears it frequently spreads to other countries before vaccine against it can be made.

Side effects and contraindications. A mild febrile reaction may be produced. The vaccine should not be given to subjects with a history of sensitivity or allergy.

Typhoid-paratyphoid vaccine

Pharmacological action. Vaccines containing killed Salmonella typhi with components of paratyphoid A and B are used. There is no doubt as to the effectiveness of the vaccines containing the salmonella typhi, but the value of the paratyphoid components is doubtful. With a potent vaccine immunity lasts for 3–5 years.

Therapeutic use. The vaccine is given by deep subcutaneous or intra-muscular injection. The first dose is 0·25 ml, and the second dose given after an interval of 7 to 28 days is 0·5 ml depending on the manu-facturer's instructions. In areas where the disease is prevalent reinforc-ing (booster) doses should be given every three years.

Side effects and contraindications. Reaction rates are high, with pain and/or swelling at the site of injection, chills and fever several hours after administration, myalgia, arthralgia, nausea and occasional vomiting.

Diphtheria toxoid

Pharmacological action. The toxoid is prepared from the toxin which ap-pears in a culture of Corynebacterium diphtheriae. A very high degree of protection is provided.

Therapeutic use [7]. The toxoid is sometimes given together with tetanus toxoid. The basic course of immunisation comprises three injections, at intervals of 4 to 8 weeks between the first and second, and 6 to 12 months between the second and third. Booster doses of diphtheria toxoid are given only in certain armed forces and where there is a high risk of exposure to infection, e.g. among nurses in fever hospitals.

Side effects. Occasionally there is tenderness at the site of injection. Very rarely immunisation may be complicated by a general reaction (head-ache, vomiting, and malaise). These symptoms are transient.

The only serious hazard has been that of 'provocation poliomyelitis' developing in the limb into which the diphtheria antigen has been infected. This risk has been minimised by the general use of polio-myelitis vaccination.

References

1. Kaplan, C., *Brit. med. Bull.* (1969), **25**, 131.
2. Harrison, T. R., *Principles of Internal Medicine* (1966), McGraw-Hill, New York, 1720.
3. Turner, G. S., *Brit. med. Bull.* (1969), **25**, 136.
4. Beale, A. J., *ibid,* 148.
5. Rees, R. J. W., *ibid,* 183.
6. Tyrrell, D. A. J., *ibid,* 165.
7. Ellis, R. W. B., and Mitchell, R. G., *Disease in Infancy and childhood* (1968), 551, Livingstone, London.

This chapter was written by Dr P. I. Folb (Dept of Clinical Pharmacology, Guy's Hospital Medical School) and edited by Prof. J. R. Trounce.

Supplement

DRUG INTERACTION

With ever-increasing numbers of potent agents available for prescription and simultaneous administration the problem of drug interaction is becoming a very serious one. And these interactions are not merely theoretical possibilities. Even now there is a large number of potentially dangerous effects that may be produced by the interaction of commonly used and necessary drugs [1, 2]. Interaction may occur at any site along the pathway from administration to excretion and occasionally even before the drugs are given. A classification of such interactions is appended (modified from Herxheimer, 1969 see [1]) with in addition a list of some of the more important drugs implicated.

1. *Before administration.* E.g. suxamethonium and thiopentone react chemically in solution.

2. *At the site of entry.* E.g. the chelating effect of oral tetracyclines on calcium and aluminium in the gut.

3. *Interaction during binding to blood or tissue proteins.* Many acidic drugs bind to plasma albumin, e.g. phenylbutazone, warfarin, clofibrate and sulphonamides and any two of these drugs may compete for this binding giving an abnormally high free plasma concentration of the drug which has the least affinity for the binding sites. A similar situation has been described for tissue proteins in relation to antimalarial therapy. Less often a drug will increase its binding to protein in the presence of another drug, e.g. pempidine and chlorothiazide [3].

4. *At the site of action.* E.g. isoprenaline and propranolol; folic acid and methotrexate, etc.

5. *During metabolism.* Here interactions are usually effected by inhibition or stimulation of drug metabolizing enzymes, e.g. barbiturates, antiepileptics and phenylbutazone are all potent stimulators of the liver microsomal enzymes which are responsible for the metabolism of these and other drugs, e.g. chloramphenicol, M.A.O. inhibitors and methylphenidate, see [4]. M.A.O. inhibitors, however, are better known for their inactivation of mono-amine oxidase and the potentiation of amines, such as tyramine, present in high quantities in certain foods.

6. *During excretion.* Competition may occur between drugs requiring the same pathway for excretion, e.g. probenicid and peni-

cillin. The excretion of weakly acidic or weakly basic drugs may be affected by agents that modify the urinary pH and therefore the degree of ionisation and tubular reabsorption.

Particular interactions to note

PHENYLBUTAZONE, SULPHONAMIDES, CLOFIBRATE and SALICYLATES may seriously potentiate the effect of oral anti-coagulants, e.g. WARFARIN, due to its displacement from binding to serum albumin. Similarly, SALICYLATES may potentiate the effect of SULPHONAMIDES, SULPHONYL UREAS and METHO-TREXATE. BARBITURATES reduce the effect of many drugs by stimulating the metabolising enzymes in the liver, and the drugs affected include, once again, the oral anticoagulants.

When the interaction produces a *reduced* effect the potentially serious consequences may not be realised until the inhibiting drug such as a barbiturate is stopped (e.g. on leaving hospital) and a previously well-controlled patient on an oral anticoagulant goes out of control. In addition to the barbiturates, glutethimide, dichloralphenazone and several other drugs also have this effect [5]. It may be that other non-barbiturate hypnotics cause much less stimulation of these enzymes, but much work still needs to be done to clarify this point. By quite a different mechanism barbiturates potentiate the effects of alcohol on the central nervous system.

M.A.O. INHIBITORS and METHYLPHENIDATE will increase the plasma concentration and effect of such drugs as BARBITURATES, most ANTIEPILEPTIC AGENTS and ORAL ANTICOAGULANTS by inhibiting drug metabolism.

It is obvious that therapeutic anticoagulation with oral agents (e.g. with warfarin or phenindione) may be disturbed by a variety of drug interactions. The mechanism of these is summarised in the table on the next page.

M.A.O. INHIBITORS will interact with AMINES of all kinds often with serious effects. TRICYCLIC antidepressants antagonise the hypotensive effects of ADRENERGIC blocking agents, see [9].

PROPRANOLOL may not only potentiate the hypoglycaemic effect of INSULIN but also masks the warning symptoms of sweating and tachycardia. PENTAZOCINE like other narcotic antagonists may precipitate a withdrawal syndrome in those physically dependent on other analgesics.

A comprehensive review of this subject has recently appeared [10]

Drug Interaction and Anticoagulation

Mechanism	Examples of drugs implicated	Effect on Anticoagulation	References
1. Reduction in absorption of Vitamin K.	Oral liquid paraffin	Increased	[6]
2. Alteration of gut flora with reduced local synthesis of Vitamin K.	Broad spectrum antibiotics	Increased	[6]
3. Diarrhoea with increased loss of anticoagulant in the stools.	Broad spectrum antibiotics	Reduced	[6]
4. Decreased plasma albumin binding.	Phenylbutazone, salicylates, etc.	Increased	[7]
5. Increased drug metabolism.	Barbiturates, etc.	Reduced	[8]
6. Decreased drug metabolism.	M.A.O. inhibitors, methylphenidate, etc.	Increased	[4]

and an awareness of the general lines along which these interactions occur may help to reduce their incidence. Some drugs may interact by more than one mechanism, e.g. sulphonamides and sulphonyl ureas cause an effect both on plasma albumin binding and on drug metabolising enzymes. Nevertheless the basic point is that they interact and this is what should be remembered.

DRUGS AND RENAL FAILURE

A large number of drugs are excreted by the kidney and in renal failure accumulation of these drugs may occur. Under these circumstances smaller doses will be required. The dose can be determined (a) on an *ad hoc* basis, by observing the clinical response of the patient; (b) by repeated measurement of blood levels, if this is possible; or (c) by measuring the glomerular filtration rate and by calculation of the reduction in excretion which will occur. This latter method is only possible when the mode of excretion of the drug is known.

In general terms when a drug is largely excreted by glomerular filtration no reduction of dosage is required if the GFR is above 30 ml/min. If the GFR is between 15–30 ml/min, two-thirds of the dose is required and if it is below 15 ml/min, one-third of the dose is required.

Antibiotics

1. The penicillins and cephaloridine are largely excreted by the kidney though in renal failure a certain amount is excreted by other routes, probably the liver.

2. Streptomycin, kanamycin, gentamycin. Great care is needed with these drugs as ototoxicity is a real risk. If possible blood levels should be estimated.

3. Tetracyclines are partially excreted via the kidneys and should be avoided in uraemia since they increase the blood urea.

4. Chloramphenicol is inactivated in the liver but accumulation of metabolities of possible toxicity can occur.

5. Fucidic acid and oleandomycin do not depend on renal clearance.

Narcotics – These are not excreted by the kidney.

Hypnotics and sedatives

Phenothiazines and barbiturates are partially excreted by the kidney. Long-acting barbiturates (such as phenobarbitone) are particularly likely to accumulate.

Diazepam and chlordiazepoxide are entirely metabolised and no reduced dose is required.

Cardiovascular drugs

Digoxin is partially excreted by the kidney and smaller doses are required.

Procainamide is about 50 per cent excreted in the urine and lignocaine largely excreted by the kidney.

Most blood pressure lowering drugs are partially or wholly excreted by the kidney with the possible exception of reserpine.

References

1. Herxheimer, A., *Prescribers' Journal* (1969), **9**, 62.
2. Launchbury, A. P., A table of some drug (and other) interactions. Initially published February 1966 in *J. Hosp. Pharm.*, **23**, 24, and later revised and

published separately by Thomas Waide and Sons, Kirkstall Hall, Leeds, P.O. Box 140, England.

3. Dollery, C. T., Emslie-Smith, D., and Muggleton, P. G., *Proc. Roy. Soc. Med.* (1960), **53**, 592.

4. Garrettson, L. K., Perel, K. M., and Dayton, P. G., *J.A.M.A.* (1969), **207**, 2053.

5. Breckenridge, A., Orme, M. L'E., Davies, D. S., and Thorgeirsson, S., *Clin. Sci.* (1969), **37**, 565.

6. Editors: Goodman, L. S. and Gilman, A. *The Pharmacological basis of therapeutics* (1966), Third Edition, pages 1453-4, Macmillan.

7. Aggeler, P. M., O'Reilly, R. A., Leong, L., and Kowitz, P. E., *New Eng. J. Med.* (1967), **276**, 496.

8. Burns, J. J., Cucinell, S. A., Koster, R., and Conney, A. H., *Ann. N.Y. Acad. Sci.* (1965), **123**, 273.

9. Skinner, C., Coull, D. C., and Johnston, A. W., *Lancet* (1969), **ii**, 564.

10. Prescott, L. F., *Lancet* (1969), **ii**, 1239.

Index

Index